Advances for Prosthetic Technology

Robert LeMoyne

Advances for Prosthetic Technology

From Historical Perspective to Current Status to Future Application

Springer

Robert LeMoyne
Department of Biological Sciences
Northern Arizona University
Flagstaff
Arizona
USA

ISBN 978-4-431-55814-9 ISBN 978-4-431-55816-3 (eBook)
DOI 10.1007/978-4-431-55816-3

Library of Congress Control Number: 2015951821

Springer Tokyo Heidelberg New York Dordrecht London

Printed on acid-free paper

Springer Japan KK is part of Springer Science+Business Media (www.springer.com)

To my wife, thank you for everything. Love Always.
I would like to thank my Mother, Father, and brother for their support.
"Nothing transcends the power of the human spirit."
from a homeless Vietnam Veteran and very loyal friend
And in the wind he's still alive.
"To beat a tiger, one needs a brother's help."
Chinese Proverb
Thanks Tim.
"Chiri mo tsumoreba yama to naru."
A favorite Japanese Proverb (in Romaji)
Translation:
"Even dust piled up becomes a mountain."

Preface

To be an effective research and development engineer for the domain of the transtibial powered prostheses, one needs a broad knowledge base, creativity, and compassion. The objective of this book is to encompass multiple fields of discipline that in consideration of each chapter could literally barely touch upon entire fields of medical and engineering specialties toward which people can dedicate their career. The understanding of the true nature of the complexities that constitute the foundation for gait with respect to the ankle–foot complex is rapidly growing.

The powered prosthesis is inherently a mechatronic system with many supporting subsystems, such as through an actuator, control, and sensors. Software also encompasses a considerable foundation for the optimal design. As the domain of mechatronics is growing at an effectively exponential rate, the opportunities for future powered prostheses are expected to grow. Each powered prosthetic configuration can provide a unique design objective for the person with amputation who uses that specific device.

Creativity is a ubiquitous skill developed over the life evolution of a diligent engineer/scientist. With respect to compassion, transtibial powered prostheses must be realized not as a complex mechatronic device to boast of one's skill and brilliance regarding its progressive development. The transtibial powered prosthesis will be used by a person with an amputation for thousands of steps a day. The prosthesis will restore a person to a preferred level of personally unique activity, giving back a semblance of that simple joy of something that was once taken.

Flagstaff, AZ — Robert LeMoyne

Contents

Chapter 1
Amputations and Prostheses, a Topic of Global Concern

Abstract A preliminary comprehensive overview of the role of the prothesis, in particular the transtibial prosthesis is presented. With the increasing number of people experiencing amputation, there is considerable motivation to advance the technology capabilities of the lower limb prosthesis. The historical origins of the prosthesis are presented from a diversity of geographic perspectives. A general historic perspective of the evolutionary trends from passive to energy storage and return that lead to the modern powered prostheses are established with the pathway leading to the state of the art powered prosthesis. The diverse fields of engineering that support the research and development of prosthetic technology are emphasized. A brief preview of the basis for amputation, amputation surgical procedure evolution, and post-amputation surgery are amended to provide a global perspective. The role of functional classification scales for the purpose of identifying rehabilitation status are discussed. In summary, a broad series of subjects provide the evolutionary basis for the improvement of prostheses serving to better the quality of life for people with amputation.

Keywords Prosthetic evolutionary trends • Basis for amputation • Amputation surgical procedure • Functional classification • Post-amputation surgery

1.1 Introduction

The growing prevalence of amputation is driving the need to evolve, research, and develop supporting technology for the domain of the prosthesis. For example developed countries, such as the United States of America, the United Kingdom, and Germany are experiencing notable levels of amputations relative to their populations (Ziegler-Graham et al. 2008; Grimmer and Seyfarth 2014). Especially in the United States of America, approximately one-million people have experienced lower limb amputation. Based on recent projections, the number of people with amputation by 2050 is anticipated to double (Ziegler-Graham et al. 2008; Grabowski and D'Andrea 2013). Based on these observations, there is an imperative motivation to substantially advance the technology domain of the prosthesis.

However, the scope of the technology advance must also address the economic capabilities of a diversity of nations. Consider the developing nation of Vietnam.

R. LeMoyne, *Advances for Prosthetic Technology*,
DOI 10.1007/978-4-431-55816-3_1

Advanced technology prosthesis ubiquitous to the ecosystem of a developed country, such as a nation of the G8, may not be viable for a developing economy. Currently, the International Committee of the Red Cross estimates the manufacturing cost of polypropylene prostheses to be below the threshold of $100 (Coupland 1997). In such a case, more economically robust alternatives may be attractive.

The surgical domain of amputations can span from limbs of the upper body (arms) and lower body (legs) at any level. The nature of the amputation is generally denoted according to the predominant bone at the level of the amputation. A transhumeral amputation occurs at the level of the upper arm. A transradial amputation pertains to the lower arm. With regards to the lower limbs a transfemoral amputation occurs at the upper leg. A transtibial amputation occurs between the ankle and knee (May and Lockard 2011).

The objective of this book is to provide a comprehensive perspective regarding the transtibial prosthesis with an emphasis on restoration of walking functionality. The removal of the ankle-foot complex imparts many issues for a person's gait, with many physiological implications regarding amputation. Asymmetry of gait and compensatory strategies intuitively can develop with the adaptation to a transtibial prosthesis. These perturbations from natural gait can lead to long-term morbidities. Gait analysis techniques, such as biomechanical analysis, are foundational for the establishment of improved prosthetic technologies. There are many classes of transtibial prostheses, such as the traditional passive prosthesis, recent passive prosthesis with energy storage and return, and novel state of the art powered prosthesis (LeMoyne 2015). These topics are addressed throughout the book with an emphasis from a system-based perspective. A historic perspective on the evolution of the prosthesis is essential for addressing the state of the art.

1.2 The Evolution of the Prosthesis, from Historic Origins to Modern Technology

The origins of the prosthesis derive from a geographic diversity of advanced civilizations, such as India, Egypt, Greece, and Rome. Preliminary applications were oriented both toward restoration of function and cosmetic appearance (Duraiswami et al. 1971; LeMoyne 2015). Based on transcripts dated on the order of four millennia, there is documentation of a Queen within the region of India surviving an amputation, later to be fitted with a prosthesis made of iron. This ancient prosthetic leg enabled her to walk and return to the battlefield (Duraiswami et al. 1971). The ancient civilization of Egypt developed prostheses with the objective of improving function and appearance (Hernigou 2013; LeMoyne 2015). The Romans and the Greeks advanced prostheses for the intent of rehabilitation (Thurston 2007; Hernigou 2013; LeMoyne 2015).

During the 1500's, a transformative innovator of the lower limb prosthesis was Ambroise Paré. A surgeon for the French Army, Paré lived from 1510 to

1590. The prostheses developed by Paré resembled modern prostheses for the lower limb. For example, Paré produced a prosthesis that incorporated modern design characteristics, such as an articulated joint about the knee and an emulation of a prosthetic foot for structural purposes (Thurston 2007; May and Lockard 2011; Hernigou 2013; LeMoyne 2015).

Pieter Adriaanszoon Verduyn of Holland and James Potts of England advanced further developments of industrial-era lower leg prostheses. During 1696 Verduyn demonstrated a transtibial prosthesis capable of unlocking at the knee joint. Potts in 1843 created a lower limb prosthesis with the functional capacity to provide dorsiflexion, which involves the orienting the toe toward the tibia. This feature was enabled though flexing at the knee joint. Potts' prosthesis consisted of materials representative of that era, such as steel, leather, and wood (May and Lockard 2011).

The concept of the prosthesis eventually permeated distant countries, such as Japan. Neighboring nations, such as China, influenced Japanese medicine. However, with the introduction of European medical standards, the concept of the prosthesis constituted a paradigm shift. For example, translations of the works of Ambroise Paré eventual reached Japan during the 1700s (Takechi 1992).

The first Japanese citizen to use a prosthesis was Tanosuke Sawamura III a famous Kabuki actor during the late 1860s. Similar to Western nations, a primary driver for Japan's development of prosthetic technology was for the treatment of their soldiers as a consequence of war. As a consequence of a shortage of raw materials following the Second World War, Japan innovated the concept of using indigenous bamboo for aspects of the lower limb prosthesis, such as for a basket socket and pylon. In alignment with Japan's significant economic development, considerable research and development achievements have been established (Takechi 1992).

The American Civil War from 1861 to 1865 induced progress regarding technological improvements and government-level policy advances for persons with amputations. During the Civil War the United State Congress passed legislation providing free prostheses for veterans who lost limbs as a consequence of war. One veteran in particular J.E. Hanger founded his own company with the mission of advancing prostheses. As a survivor of a leg amputation, one of his inventions was the incorporation of a rubber bumper about the ankle to emulate better control about the prosthetic representation of the ankle-foot complex (May and Lockard 2011).

Research and development thrusts for advances in prostheses have been accelerated as a consequence of warfare and the obligation of a nation to ameliorate the disabilities for veterans with amputation. The broad scale of the two world wars of the last century has established such motivation. National institutions have sponsored and supported research and development initiatives for modern prosthetic technologies (Thurston 2007; May and Lockard 2011; Hernigou 2013; LeMoyne 2015).

During the end of the Second World War the Surgeon General for the Army of the United States of America issued request for counsel from the National Academy of Sciences regarding the provision prostheses for the considerable number of soldiers who survived amputation. The findings, consisting of the recommendation from prosthetists, surgeons, and engineers, advised the initiation of research for advancing prosthetic applications. The National Academy of Sciences instituted a Committee on Prosthetics Research and Development. The committee predominantly consisted of prosthetists, engineers, and physicians, which directed broad research and development for a considerable scope in conjunction with multiple public and private institutions. Two accomplishments of the research endeavors for the scope of transtibial amputation are the patellar tendon bearing socket and the Solid Ankle Cushioned Heel (SACH) (Wilson 1963).

Exponential growth of the global domain of prosthetic technologies has occurred since the 1970s. Improved comprehension of the foundation of human gait has been elucidated. Materials have advanced enabling lighter weight structural components. Microprocessors, software, and sensors enable advanced prostheses to function as adaptable and intelligent robotic systems. The modern prosthesis draws upon from diverse fields of science and engineering, such as biomedical engineering, mechanical engineering, electrical engineering, robotic engineering, and computer science (Thurston 2007; May and Lockard 2011; Hernigou 2013; LeMoyne 2015).

The modern transtibial prosthesis spans three domains of system applications. The SACH prosthesis emphasizes the role of providing structural support, such as during the general stance phase of gait. However, the need for restoring an amount of the energy initially imparted during stance has led to the development of the Energy Storage and Return (ESAR) prosthesis. Some versions of this class are passive regarding energy return, and others are equipped with mechanisms to provide controlled energy return (May and Lockard 2011; LeMoyne 2015).

Within roughly the past decade, transtibial prostheses have been developed that function as a mechatronic robotic system that intelligently adjusts to various phases of the gait cycle. These prosthetic systems incorporate state of the art actuator technology, software, and sensors to provide the user with maximal restorative function during gait, such as additional mechanical energy to the terminal aspects of the stance phase of gait (May and Lockard 2011; LeMoyne 2015). One of the pioneers of this class of robotic powered prosthesis is Dr. Hugh Herr who leads the MIT Media Lab's Biomechatronics research group (Herr). Dr. Herr like J.E. Hanger is the survivor of lower limb amputation.

The evolutionary pathway of prosthetic technology entails a growing significance and exciting future for those who wish to commit themselves to the venerable task of restoring functionality for people with amputation. From a systems perspective advance in the supporting technologies is highly diverse with influence of many fields of engineering and science. Another important foundation for the role of advances in prostheses, such as at the transtibial level, is the motivation for amputation from a medical perspective including surgical techniques.

1.3 Motivations for Amputation and Surgical Techniques

Tandem to the evolution of prosthetic technology is the improvement in the quality of amputation surgery, which inherently correlates with the quality of a person with amputation's rehabilitation and recovery. Over the course of many centuries surgical technique for amputation have progressively evolved. These advances lead toward the capacity to prepare the residual limb with the objective of functional restoration. There exists an intrinsic relationship between the characteristics of the post-operative residual limb and the person's prosthetic socket, which is especially relevant for the long term quality of life (May and Lockard 2011).

For example, consider the inherent repetitive load bearing nature of gait. A residual limb after an amputation is an immediate result of a surgical procedure, not the musculoskeletal system resultant of evolution for human gait. The residual limb is subject to cyclical loading about soft tissue (Silver-Thorn et al. 1996; LeMoyne 2015).

The two World Wars of the twentieth century particularly perpetuated the need to improve amputation surgery. During the First World War amputations on the order of 100,000 for soldiers resulted in advances regarding the amputation level and skin flap that covers the amputation site. Surgical techniques further improved during the era of the Second World War (May and Lockard 2011).

A fundamental objective of the modern surgical procedure for amputation is to preserve as much of the residual limb as feasible. However, practical constraints exist, such as enabling the residual limb to tolerate inherent stressors and gait associated prosthetic ambulation. The level of amputation significantly affects the associated musculature and soft tissue (May and Lockard 2011).

Two surgical strategies impact the musculature that has had its distal insertion severed by the amputation: myoplasty and myodesis. The more standard myoplasty involves the attaching the musculature's anterior and posterior aspects to each other over the terminal section of the amputated bone. Myodesis is a relatively more rare surgical procedure, as it requires a more protracted duration. This procedure consists of anchoring the muscle to the bone (May and Lockard 2011).

Regarding a closed amputation procedure, there are several types of skin flap techniques available to close the site of amputation. A strategy for conserving bone length involves equal length anterior and posterior skin flaps. In the event that more distal padding is preferred, a surgeon can incorporate a long posterior flap. For severe dysvascular scenarios skew sagittal flaps can be applied, for which skew flaps utilize an anterior-posterior incision. Another strategy particularly incorporated in transtibial amputation is the development of a bony bridge between the fibula and tibia, which are amputated in a manner to establish length equivalence. The goal of this surgical technique is to enable optimal sensory feedback and prosthetic control (May and Lockard 2011).

1.4 Post-amputation Surgery

A critical aspect of a person's adaptation to an active lifestyle is the quality of the transtibial amputation. Also the length of the residual limb signifies a significant role in the nature of the rehabilitation process. Frequently amputations are conducted in less than optimal circumstances. As an amputation is a specialized procedure, a surgeon uniquely skilled with this technique is highly preferable. Some institutions even apply a highly multidisciplinary collaboration among multiple experts of the medical community, such as prosthetists, orthopedic surgeons, physical medicine specialists, and even plastic surgeons (Schnur and Meier 2014).

In the event that a rehabilitation team judges that a revision of the residual limb would enhance function and fitting of the prosthesis, further post-operative surgery may be advised. Some conditions warranting revision surgery may only become apparent during the acute phase of rehabilitation and recovery:

- The presence of sharp bony protrusions that induce pain while wearing the socket of the prosthesis
- Insufficient coverage of soft-tissue
- Inadequate contouring of the residual limb
- Heterotopic bone formation that causes discomfort about the socket
- Formation of a neuroma (Schnur and Meier 2014)

As inferred by the progressively evolving nature of some of these scenarios, a person with an amputation may be compelled for revisional surgery as a result of their residual limb undergoing a non-optimal healing pattern.

More advanced techniques that would require residual limb revision have been implemented in other levels of amputation. Targeted muscle reinnervation has been applied for upper limb prosthetic applications that utilize the subject's neural signal. In order to make such a prosthesis feasible the neural pathway is revised by surgical intervention (Schnur and Meier 2014).

Another technique is osseous integration, which involves direct skeletal attachment of the prosthetic socket interface. Prosthetic suspension that features osseointegrated implants constitutes a paradigm shift from the traditional socket suspension. This technique is envisioned to facilitate load transfer between the residual limb and prosthesis as forces are applied directly to the skeletal structure rather than a soft tissue interface with sensory afferent representation (Schnur and Meier 2014).

In the event that the preliminary residual limb is too short a bone lengthening procedure may be warranted. A short residual limb can impair ambulation with reduced leverage and can also provide insufficient surface area to distribute forces about the prosthetic interface. Bone lengthening can be applied through an allograft of cadaver bone to provide more appropriate leverage to ambulate the prosthesis (Schnur and Meier 2014).

Post-amputation operations have been developed for the goal of better stabilizing the transected tibia and fibula. As described in Chap. 2: 'Ankle-foot complex and the fundamental aspects of gait' that elucidates the intricate anatomy of the ankle-foot complex, the tibia and fibula are interconnected at the distal ends of both bones. Transtibial amputation induces tibiofibular instability as the tibia and fibula are only attached at the superior aspect not the level of the amputation (Lewandowski et al. 2013). As the distal end of a transtibial amputation residual limb is not designed for load bearing, considerable discomfort can arise (LeMoyne 2015). Such a degree of discomfort and even pain may challenge progress regarding rehabilitation.

During 1949 Dr. Etrl innovated a technique still implemented as of current, now know as the Etrl procedure. Dr. Ertl developed a procedure for constructing a bone bridge between the tibia and fibula. Over time a U-shape bone structure would ossify, which would facilitate a better weight bearing capacity relative to a separate tibia and fibula configuration (Ertl 1949; Pinto and Harris 2004). Other newer techniques have propose utilizing a fibular segment to induce synostosis between the tibia and fibula (Pinto and Harris 2004).

1.5 Functional Classification of Rehabilitation Status

In the medical community ordinal scales are applied to define a subject's status of rehabilitation. For people with amputation, a five-point ordinal scale has been established as a prognosticator for forecasting rehabilitation potential. The ordinal scale requires a skilled clinician, such as a prosthetist, to subjectively evaluate a patient relative to series of criteria ratings. Based on the expert interpretation of the clinician, the patient's state of rehabilitation is assigned to an appropriate ordinal level (May and Lockard 2011).

The benefit of the ordinal scale methodology is for the conveyance of a patient's rehabilitation status throughout the medical community. A subject's state of recovery can be conveyed to medical insurance for compensation of prosthetic components. Also since this approach is recognized throughout the medical community, a subject's ordinal scale ranking can provide acuity for new clinicians regarding the patients treatment. Medicare (an American institution) has developed functional classification levels, which are referred to as K-level, which consists of five ordinal points ranging from 0 to 4 (May and Lockard 2011):

0. At functional level 0 a prosthesis is considered as not improving a patient's mobility or quality of life. This scenario entails a patient lacking the potential or capability to safely ambulate even with assistance.
1. Functional level 1 characterizes a patient capable of limited and unlimited ambulation in a household environment. This classification is representative of a patient that can ambulate on level surfaces with cadence that is fixed.
2. Function level 2 describes a patient that is able to conduct limited ambulation in the patient's community. This level entails the ability to traverse environmental barriers, such as uneven surfaces, stairs, and curbs.

3. At functional level 3 the constraints for simple locomotion are exceeded with the capability or potential to conduct ambulation at variable cadence. The patient is also able to transcend most environmental barriers.
4. At function level 4 people with an amputation is characterized as an active adult or athlete. The thresholds for basic ambulation proficiencies are surpassed (May and Lockard 2011).

Another ordinal scale classifier to identify mobility for a person with lower limb amputation is the Special Interest Group in Amputee Medicine (SIGAM). The SIGAM scale is envisioned to determine changes regarding mobility. The SIGAM scale is comprised of six ordinal components. The application of the SIGAM scale involves answering a series of 21 questions representing a comprehensive mobility questionnaire. An algorithm is then applied to the responses, and the appropriate SIGAM grade is ascertained. The six grade levels are characterized by the following descriptions:

A. The purpose of the prosthesis is for cosmetic use or abandoned entirely.
B. The prosthesis is used primarily for facilitating mobility with another person assisting or for therapy.
C. The user of the prosthesis is capable of walking on a level surface for less than 50 m with or without an assistive device.
D. The subject can walk in excess of 50 m on a level surface with good outdoor weather conditions with or without an assistive device.
E. The subject can walk for greater than 50 m without an assistive device. The occasion of using an assistive device is generally restrained to severe weather or terrain conditions.
F. The subject exhibits gait capabilities at parity or near parity to people without amputation (Ryall et al. 2003).

Such functional classification levels are not only relevant and useful to solely the clinical community. These classifications are also pertinent to the prosthetic research and development community, since coherent testing and evaluating of subjects at similar functional classification levels permits congruence of research findings (LeMoyne 2015). For example Mancinelli et al. developed a research study that applied people classified at SIGAM grade E and F, in order to emphasize people with high level ambulation (Mancinelli et al. 2011).

1.6 Preprosthetic Activity Level and Chapter Perspectives

A person's activity level prior to a transtibial amputation is an important indicator for the prediction of post-ambutation rehabilitation and recovery. A person with an active and independent lifestyle is highly likely to be strongly motivated to return to such a quality of life after adapting to a prosthesis. Many factors influence the quality of prosthetic training and functional outcomes, such as the following considerations:

- The person's ability to return to an active lifestyle during the healing timeframe of the residual limb
- Involvement in an exercise (therapy) regiment that sustains strength and mitigates contractures
- Keeping ambulatory even with a provisional prosthesis inclusive of reduced weight bearing (May and Lockard 2011)

The correlation between a person's lifestyle prior to amputation surgery and subsequent quality of life while adapting to a prosthesis has been identified a topic of minimal research (May and Lockard 2011).

Further investigation into this matter of pre-operative activity and post-operative adaptation may better elucidate a person with amputation's functional outcome throughout the rehabilitation process. The following factors have been identified as influential toward the realization of function outcome goals:

- Activity level from a premorbid perspective
- Activity level from a preprosthetic perspective
- Amputation level
- Comorbidities influencing physical stamina and balance
- Nature of the injury or disease that escalated to a amputation
- Correlation between the quality of prosthetic components to functional aptitudes
- Extent of contractures with regards to the hip flexor musculature (May and Lockard 2011)

Post-amputation procedures exist for the improvement of the quality of life of people with an amputation in order to enable their functional goals more attainable (May and Lockard 2011).

As amputation surgery techniques have improved, other fields that strongly influence prosthetic technology have progressively evolved. Gait analysis technology and the comprehension of the ankle-foot complex anatomy have better elucidated the nature of gait for people with transtibial amputation. Over three and a half decades transtibial prosthesis have evolved considerably from passive prostheses that provide primarily structural support to passive prosthesis that contribute a degree of energy storage and return during gait. Recently with multiple advances in robotic technology, especially at the actuator and control level, powered prostheses capable of providing positive work to gait have been realized (LeMoyne 2015).

As this book shall imply each topic addressed for each chapter can literally be expanded into a book itself. The subject of providing meaningful prosthetic technology for people with amputation spans a considerable number of fields and expertise. For example the ankle-foot complex is applicable to an entire field of medicine known a podiatry. Neurology establishes the foundation for gait control. Gait analysis is the domain of the kinesiologist and physical therapist. The current thrust of prosthetic technology emphasizes the development of robust powered prostheses, which spans multiple diverse engineering fields, such as biomedical engineering, mechanical engineering, electrical engineering, and computer science.

The objective of this book is to elucidate the multiple fields that encompass the development of substantive prosthesis for people with transtibial amputation. An emphasis is placed on the evolutionary foundations for developing powered prostheses and their current implementations.

The book is organized into the following chapters:

Chapter 2: "Ankle-foot complex and the fundamental aspects of gait"

The objective of this chapter is to underscore the intricacy of the ankle-foot complex. As demonstrated by prostheses of the prior to roughly the mid twentieth century, the transtibial prosthesis primarily served a structural role. The ankle-foot complex entails a multi-disciplinary function with regards to musculo-skeletal and neurological capabilities. These attributes integrate toward the fluid and synchronous gait functionality. Intuitively a transected ankle-foot complex necessitates the development of a powered prosthesis that satisfies a multitude of requirements. The comprehension of the role of the ankle-foot complex for gait, especially for the stance phase, is imperative for the modern design of powered prosthetic systems. With the significance of the ankle-foot complex summarized the general characteristics of the standard gait cycle emphasizing the status of the ankle-foot complex are defined. A global perspective of the role of the ankle-foot complex and its inherent contribution to gait are imperative for a research team seeking to develop a meaningful evolution of powered prosthetic technology for people with transtibial amputation.

Chapter 3: "Prosthetic gait asymmetry and discomfort while walking with a transtibial prosthesis"

The challenges a person with a transtibial amputation must handle are a subject of this chapter. Asymmetry about the gait likely can develop. As gait is highly repetitive, especial for those desiring to maintain an active lifestyle, the considerable number of steps per day may induce morbidities, such as arthritis and atrophy patterns. With the lack of natural powered plantar flexion about the residual limb, a person with a lower limb amputation can expend amplified metabolic energy, which can even impact and diminish the optimal walking speed. With a better understanding of induced asymmetry during gait an engineering research and development team can better serve their customer (people with lower limb amputation) with a superior powered prosthesis.

Chapter 4: "Testing and evaluation strategies for the powered prosthesis, a global perspective"

In order to address the efficacy of a prosthetic research and development endeavor an understanding of the biomechanics of gait is significant. This chapter intends to provide the reader with a introductory perspective regarding biomechanical analysis of gait. Equipment used to conduct gait analysis is also discussed. With the knowledge elucidated, ideally a group could assemble a preliminary gait laboratory. Associated procedures inherent with experimental techniques, such as prosthetic alignment and subject inclusion criteria, are presented. Advanced concepts that are relevant to the domain of gait analysis, such as machine learning and mobile gait platforms (smartphones), are covered as topics of interest.

Chapter 5: "Passive transtibial prosthesis and associated prosthetic components"

After the Second World War an American multi-institutional research and development endeavor advanced transtibial prosthetic technology with the Solid Ankle Cushioned Heel (SACH). Although many new types of prostheses have been developed since, the SACH is robust, inexpensive, and may still provide considerable application specific utility. This chapter also emphasizes the integral nature of a transtibial prosthetic system. For example, the socket, liner, suspension, and pylon all serve critical function to the overall utility of many types of prosthesis. In essence, a design team could theoretically assemble a well engineered powered prosthesis, but a deficiency with regards to the socket, liner, suspension, and pylon could cause a person with an amputation considerable discomfort.

Chapter 6: "Energy Storage and Return (ESAR) prosthesis"

As the role of powered plantar flexion was better comprehended during the 1980s, prosthetic designers developed prostheses that can store and return energy. These prostheses are known as Energy Storage And Return (ESAR). A portion of the energy is stored during the preliminary aspect of stance and released during the terminal phase of stance. This class of prosthesis is well used among people with amputation desiring an active lifestyle. A notable issue is that the timing of the energy release is not controlled. Further evolution of this concept has resulted in the Controlled Energy Storage and Return (CESR). The controlled release is regulated by a mechatronic system that governs the timing of the release of the stored potential energy about the terminal aspect of stance.

Chapter 7: "Architecture of a powered prosthesis system: actuators, sensors, and control"

In order to understand the foundation for a powered prosthesis, this chapter is dedicated to its architecture. A powered prosthesis constitutes an intelligent robotic system. There are three primary levels that define the architecture: actuator, sensor, and control. The most prevalent type of actuator for powered prostheses is the series elastic actuator, and other types of actuators, such as monopropellant and pneumatic actuators, are also featured. The energy source of an electro-mechanic series elastic actuator, such as a battery, is also covered. Sensors provide afferent acuity for the control system and overall prosthetic function. General control systems used to regulate the phased nature of gait in a highly synchronous manner are examined.

Chapter 8: "Transtibial powered prostheses: single and dual actuator configurations"

Two classes of powered prosthesis are presented: single actuator power prosthesis and dual actuator power prosthesis. A multitude of single actuator powered prostheses have been developed through the endeavors of research and development teams. These powered prostheses are thoroughly discussed in this chapter. An emphasis is placed on design objectives, implementation of concepts to achieve the objectives, design, and preliminary test and evaluation. Dual actuator concepts for powered prostheses have provided an evolution in capability. Dual actuator powered prostheses have enabled multi-joint functionality, such as a segmented prosthetic foot that produces powered plantar flexion through the ankle and power contribution through the primary toe. With a dual actuator architecture, a powered prosthesis can facilitate ankle inversion and eversion, which can enhance a person with amputation's quality of life. Another exciting goal is to enable soldiers who have experienced amputation the opportunity to return to active duty with a robust dual powered prosthesis. In order to achieve this goal, which a half-century ago would have been considered incomprehensible, the dual actuator perspective serves a vital role.

Chapter 9: "The MIT inspired powered prosthesis leading to the commercialized BiOM powered prosthesis, a precedence in transtibial prosthetic technology"

The most prevalent commercial powered prosthesis for people with transtibial amputation is the iWalk BiOM. This prosthesis facilitates the user with powered plantar flexion through a detailed control system that is implemented through a well positioned sensor system. The iWalk BiOM's origins stem from research and development through the Massachusetts Institute of Technology. The evolutionary pathway of this powered prosthesis that utilizes a series elastic actuator and finite state machine is thoroughly addressed. A considerable degree of testing and evaluation has been applied to this powered prosthesis, which is also entailed in this chapter.

Chapter 10: "Future and advanced concepts for the powered prosthesis"

A perspective on future concepts for the transtibial prosthesis elucidates the near term of potential evolutions. A particular subject of interest is the development of intelligent and essentially autonomous adaptation of a transtibial prosthesis to a subject's lifestyle preferences. This trend is envisioned to provide a better prosthetic emulation to the ankle-foot complex. The Internet of Things is considered to be an instrumental capability for enabling intelligent prosthetic adaptation. Mobile sensor platforms are assumed to provide the foundation. Machine learning is forecasted to provide considerably advanced diagnostic acuity in a mobile context. Other technology trends, such as 3D printing, are presumed to serve significant roles with the personalization of a person's transtibial prosthesis.

Conclusion

In summary, there is a progressively rising trend anticipated for the number of people experiencing amputation. Advances in prosthetic technologies are imperative for improving the quality of life for people with amputation. There are multiple types of prostheses that apply to upper and lower limbs, which are characterized by the level of amputation. For people with below the knee transtibial amputation the transtibial prosthesis provides considerable restorative function. The historical evolution of the transtibial prosthesis has progressed over the course human history. The origins of the transtibial prosthesis are passive in nature with notable improvements in utility. Amputation techniques and post-amputation surgery have evolved and facilitated the benefits of a lower limb prosthesis. With functional classification methods, the rehabilitation status can be more clearly defined for more

(continued)

optimal rehabilitation. Since the 1980s the role of the ankle-foot complex has been better defined, and prostheses that store and return energy have permeated the prosthetic design space. The state of the art for the transtibial prosthesis is the powered prosthesis that generates mechanically actuated work to the gait cycle. Current endeavors for advancing prosthetic technology necessitate the contribution of multidisciplinary fields of a broad scope of science and engineering.

References

Coupland RM (1997) Assistance for victims of anti-personnel mines: needs, constraints and strategy, vol 5. International Committee of the Red Cross, Geneva, pp 1–18

Duraiswami P, Orth M, Tuli S (1971) 5000 years of orthopaedics in India. Clin Orthop Relat Res 75:269–280

Ertl J (1949) Uber amputationsstumpfe. Chirurg 20:218–224

Grabowski AM, D'Andrea S (2013) Effects of a powered ankle-foot prosthesis on kinetic loading of the unaffected leg during level-ground walking. J Neuroeng Rehabil 10:1–11

Grimmer M, Seyfarth A (2014) Mimicking human-like leg function in prosthetic limbs, chap 5. In: Artemiadis P (ed) Neuro-robotics: from brain machine interfaces to rehabilitation robotics. Springer, Dordrecht

Hernigou P (2013) Ambroise Paré IV: the early history of artificial limbs (from robotic to prostheses). Int Orthop 37:1195–1197

Herr. http://www.media.mit.edu/people/hherr

LeMoyne R (2015) Advances regarding powered prosthesis for transtibial amputation. J Mech Med Biol 15:1–34

Lewandowski LR, Tintle SM, D'Alleyrand JC, Potter BK (2013) The utilization of a suture bridge construct for tibiofibular instability during transtibial amputation without distal bridge synostosis creation. J Orthop Trauma 27:e239–e242

Mancinelli C, Patritti BL, Tropea P, Greenwald RM, Casler R, Herr H, Bonato P (2011) Comparing a passive-elastic and a powered prosthesis in transtibial amputees. Proceedings of 33rd annual international conference IEEE EMBS, Boston, pp 8255–8258

May BJ, Lockard MA (2011) Prosthetics & orthotics in clinical practice: a case study approach. FA Davis, Philadelphia

Pinto MA, Harris WW (2004) Fibular segment bone bridging in trans-tibial amputation. Prosthet Orthot Int 28:220–224

Ryall NH, Eyres SB, Neumann VC, Bhakta BB, Tennant A (2003) The SIGAM mobility grades: a new population-specific measure for lower limb amputees. Disabil Rehabil 25:833–844

Schnur D, Meier RH (2014) Amputation surgery. Phys Med Rehabil Clin N Am 25:35–43

Silver-Thorn MB, Steege JW, Childress DS (1996) A review of prosthetic interface stress investigations. J Rehabil Res Dev 33:253–266

Takechi H (1992) History of prostheses and orthoses in Japan. Prosthet Orthot Int 16:98–103

Thurston AJ (2007) Paré and prosthetics: the early history of artificial limbs. ANZ J Surg 77:1114–1119

Wilson AB Jr (1963) Prosthetics and orthotics research in the United States. Orthop Prosthet Appl J 17:152–160

Ziegler-Graham K, MacKenzie EJ, Ephraim PL, Travison TG, Brookmeyer R (2008) Estimating the prevalence of limb loss in the United States: 2005 to 2050. Arch Phys Med Rehabil 89:422–429

Chapter 2
Ankle-Foot Complex and the Fundamental Aspects of Gait

Abstract In order to comprehend the scope of a transtibial amputation and provide a person with an amputation with a truly biomimetic powered prosthesis a global perspective of the ankle-foot complex must be elucidated. Even the most obvious need for structural support while standing spans the domain of highly specialized expertise. With a preliminary perspective on the skeletal complexity presented, the musculature of the ankle-foot complex constitutes a knowledge base of considerable magnitude. A brief assessment of the evolving subject of the modeling of muscle activity is summarized. A concise presentation of the intricacy of the neurological structures that the ankle-foot complex provides is examined. Topics such as the central pattern generator with afferent and efferent pathways emanating from the ankle-foot complex are discussed. Fundamental sensory mechanisms providing proprioception, which represent the spatial perception of the human body, such as muscle spindle afferents and Golgi tendon organs are entailed regarding the intrinsic contribution of the ankle-foot complex. With the contribution of these diverse aspects of the ankle-foot complex synchronous and rhythmic features of gait are enabled. The characteristics of gait can be delineated between stance and swing. The stance phase consists of highly relevant subphases, such as controlled plantar flexion, controlled dorsiflexion, and powered plantar flexion. Understanding the substantial role of the ankle-foot complex within the context of gait is imperative for a engineering/scientific research and development team to develop a powered prosthesis with optimal utility for the user.

Keywords Skeletal structure • Muscle physiology • Neurology • Gait phases • Powered plantar flexion

2.1 Introduction

The transtibial amputation involves surgically removing an entire aspect of the lower limb inferior to the transverse plane of the site of transection. The effect of an amputation about the lower leg substantially impacts the ability to walk. The removal of skeletal presence implicates the obvious need for restoration of structure to reestablish a semblance of gait.

R. LeMoyne, *Advances for Prosthetic Technology*,
DOI 10.1007/978-4-431-55816-3_2

Historic transtibial prostheses, such as those developed by Paré and Hanger, enabled the most fundamental rehabilitation criteria of structural restoration (Thurston 2007; May and Lockard 2011; Hernigou 2013). Even the SACH developed following the Second World War constitutes an evolution of this design trend (Wilson 1963). With the rapid and substantial developments encompassing the foundation and field of gait analysis, the scope of a robust and comprehensive transtibial prosthesis that truly enables and restores a person with amputation's capacity to comfortably walk has greatly advanced (Au et al. 2007a, b; Au 2007; Au and Herr 2008).

During the late 1980s Winter discovered a significant contribution of the ankle-foot complex. Approximately 80 % of the mechanical power contributed to the gait cycle is derived from plantar flexion musculature (Winter 1983; Winter and Sienko 1988; Sanderson and Martin 1997; Dobkin 2003; LeMoyne 2015). Based on this observation in the context of amputation, the mechanical work imparted to the gait cycle is considerably disrupted, and compensatory mechanisms leading to degenerative and chronic comorbidities can develop (Burke et al. 1978; Nolan et al. 2003; Mündermann et al. 2005; Morgenroth et al. 2011, 2012; LeMoyne 2015).

From a neurological perspective, efferent and especially afferent neurology considerably influences the gait cycle (Dietz 2002; LeMoyne et al. 2011). Proprioceptive afferent feedback not only establishes the body's spatial representation, but also facilitates influence about the central pattern generator, which is an inherent neurological system that affects the smooth and synchronous rhythmicity of gait (Kandel et al. 2000; Dietz 2002; Watson et al. 2010; LeMoyne 2015). The cessation of afferent contribution to neurological structures that modulate locomotion and its transition through phases and subphases can intuitively disrupt the quality of gait.

Human locomotion as of current has not been conclusively defined. The simple task of walking encompasses myriad of highly specialized medical professions, such as the podiatrist, neurologist, kinesiologist, physical therapist, and orthopedist (just to name some). The resolution of well-defined objectives for gait rehabilitation necessitates the synergistic of contribution of multiple scientific and engineering fields.

The objective of this chapter to establish the introductory fundamentals of anatomical structures that influence gait from the perspective of the lower limb. The gait cycle and its subphases are addressed. The role of neurological structures, such as the central pattern generator and afferent input, are observed. The supporting musculoskeletal structures from the descending perspective of a transtibial amputation are described.

2.2 Skeletal Aspects of the Ankle-Foot Complex

The role of skeletal aspects is to primarily enable structural support. The lower limb is supported by two long bones. They are the tibia and fibula. The tibia is situated on the medial side of the leg. The tibia is the stronger of the two bones. Lateral to the tibia resides the fibula. The primary joints for the tibia and fibula are the knee and ankle joint. Both bones facilitate attachment points for musculature that is critical for gait (Gray 1918; Saladin 2001; Seeley et al. 2003; Marieb and Hoehn 2013).

The ankle joint is primarily comprised of three bones: the tibia, fibula, and tarsus. The tarsus is a collection of seven bones that represent the superior aspect of the ankle. The largest of this set is the calcaneus, which serves two chief roles: supporting the transmission of bodyweight to ground force and enabling a lever for calf musculature that facilitates plantar flexion. The second most prevalent bone of the tarsus set is the talus. The other fives bones are comprised of the navicular. cuboid, and cuneiform (medial, intermediate, and lateral) (Gray 1918; Saladin 2001; Seeley et al. 2003; Marieb and Hoehn 2013).

Following the tarsal bones are five metatarsus that represent all five digits. The first metatarsal bone inserts to the tibialis anterior, which permits dorsiflexion. Following the metatarsals are the phalanges. The primary digit (big toe) consists of two phalanges, and the other four digits consist of three phalanges (Gray 1918; Saladin 2001; Seeley et al. 2003; Marieb and Hoehn 2013).

In summary the foot is comprised of 26 bones. These bones support 33 joints. This complex entails in excess of 100 tendons, muscles, and ligaments (APMA). The human physiology and functional anatomy has been likened to a kinetic chain. By this perspective, dysfunction to an aspect of this kinetic chain metaphor can lead to degenerative morbidities (Clark et al. 2008). With transtibial amputation leading to the removal of the entire ankle-foot complex, the damaging effects to a person's ability to function, especially without a uniquely advanced prosthesis, can be construed.

Bones are interconnected by ligaments. Ligaments are capable of absorbing energy with gradual strain under tension (Gray 1918; Ker et al. 1987; Saladin 2001; Seeley et al. 2003; Marieb and Hoehn 2013). This bone and ligament alignment enables multiple arches about the foot, such as the antero-posterior arches (inclusive of the medial and lateral arch), the fundamental longitudinal arch, and a series of transverse arches (Gray 1918; Saladin 2001; Seeley et al. 2003; Marieb and Hoehn 2013). A significant functional role of the foot arch is to absorb energy about the stance phase of gait, which can mitigate wear and injury to other aspects of the musculoskeletal system (Gray 1918; Ker et al. 1987; Saladin 2001; Seeley et al. 2003; Marieb and Hoehn 2013).

2.3 Musculature of the Ankle-Foot Complex

Articulation about the joints of the human anatomy is governed by musculature, which is capable of contracting. There are two types of contraction: concentric and eccentric. Concentric contraction is accelerative in nature, and during concentric contraction the muscle shortens. Eccentric contraction involves lengthening of the muscle while generating less force than the source of tension (Saladin 2001; Seeley et al. 2003; Clark et al. 2008; LeMoyne et al. 2008; Marieb and Hoehn 2013;

LeMoyne 2015). For example concentric contraction of the tibialis anterior imparts torque about the ankle in the dorsiflexion (toe approaching tibia) direction, such as during the swing phase of gait. By contrast, eccentric contraction serves a decelerating function, such as the smooth transition from initial contact to foot-flat of stance phase of gait. During this aspect of walking the tibialis anterior undergoes eccentric contraction (Dobkin 2003; LeMoyne et al. 2008; LeMoyne 2015).

The comprehension of muscle physiology constitutes an entire subfield of biology. The evolution of the science that encompasses muscle modeling and morphology has been progressive. However, breakthrough discoveries have challenged conventional schemes (LeMoyne 2015).

During the 1930s A.V. Hill established a perspective on the contraction of muscle that is extensively recognized to this current time frame. Hill characterized muscle force production as dependent on three primary components. The contractile element is the source of force generation. There are two springs that accompany the contractile element: a series aligned spring and a parallel oriented spring. The contributions of Hill have provided a significant foundation for modern muscle modeling (Hill 1938; Bekey 2005).

About two decades later in the 1950s Huxley enhanced the knowledge base of muscle function with the sliding filament model. This model encompasses the actin (thin filament) and myosin (thick filament) within a sarcomere. A sarcomere is a fundamental unit of musculature that extends between two adjacent Z-disks. With the introduction of Ca^{2+} as a consequence of neural activity from an action potential, binding sites of the actin become exposed. This enables the myosin head to attach to the actin establishing a cross-bridge. The attaching myosin head exert a force along the longitudinal axis. Then adenosine triphosphate (ATP) binds about the myosin head causing detachment of the myosin head. The ATP dephosphorylates to adenosine diphosphate (ADP) yielding chemical energy, which restores the myosin head to its original position for another binding site attachment with force generation (Huxley and Niedergerke 1954; Huxley and Hanson 1954; Kandel et al. 2000; Seeley et al. 2003).

Zajac during the later 1980s muscle modeling further developed by expounding upon the correlation between muscle and tendon in terms of force generation, such as the pennation angle, which is the angle between the muscle long axis and fiber angle. The pennation angle increases as a muscle progressively shortens. The soleus represents a major plantarflexor muscle of the ankle-foot complex with a pennation angle of approximately 30° (Zajac 1989; Winter 1990). Further evolutions of Zajac's contribution have resulted in internationally accepted computational muscle models, such as OpenSim (Thelen 2003; Opensim).

Scientific progress relies on discovery and then implementation of the finding to advance the state of the art model. One issue of the above muscle model contributions is the lack of a cohesive explanation for muscle history dependence, such as force enhancement and force depression. The discovery of titin and comprehension of its significance for muscle modeling has improved the model hypothesis (LeMoyne 2015).

During the 1970s the characteristics of titin were discovered (Maruyama 1976; Wang et al. 1979; Nishikawa et al. 2012). Notably this discovery was preceded by the development of many years of established research (Nishikawa et al. 2012). Nishikawa et al. have established the Winding Filament Model with titin as a Ca^{2+} activated and potential energy mechanism to better account for muscle history dependence (Nishikawa et al. 2012, 2013; Tester et al. 2012; Yeo 2012).

A major parameter that established the role of a muscle is the physiologic cross-sectional area (PCA). The PCA is representative of the quantity of sarcomeres in parallel alignment with the muscle contraction. Two classes of muscle are parallel-fiber muscle and pennate muscle. The following equations derive physiological cross-sectional area for these muscle types:

$$Parallel - fiber\ muscle\ PCA = \frac{m}{dl}$$

$$Pennate\ muscle\ PCA = \frac{m\cos(\theta)}{dl}$$

$$PCA : physiological\ cross\ section\ area\ \left(cm^2\right)$$

$$m : muscle\ fiber\ mass\ (grams)$$

$$d : muscle\ density\ \left(\frac{grams}{cm^3}\right)$$

$$l : length\ of\ muscle\ fibers\ (cm)$$

$$\theta : pennation\ angle$$

(Winter 1990)

Regarding the ankle-foot complex, the major muscles for plantar flexion are the gastrocnemius and soleus. Regarding dorsiflexion the primary muscle is the tibialis anterior. These muscles are characterized in the following table in terms of physiological cross-sectional area in terms of ankle cross section and pennation angle as described in Table 2.1.

The tibialis anterior enables dorsiflexion. Dorsiflexion is characterized by the raising of the ankle in a manner that brings the toe closer to the tibia. The tibialis anterior originates from the upper half of the tibia and inserts to the first cuneiform bone and first metatarsal bone. Neural connection is derived from the peroneal nerve (Gray 1918; Saladin 2001; Seeley et al. 2003; Marieb and Hoehn 2013).

The gastrocnemius and soleus both facilitate plantarflexion. Plantar flexion involves moving the ankle in an orientation away from the tibia. The tibial nerve innervates both muscles. The soleus originates from the fibula and tibia. Insertion occurs through the Achilles tendon that attaches to the calcaneus. The gastrocnemius also inserts to the Achilles tendon connecting to the calcaneus. However, the origin of the gastrocnemius is to the medial and lateral condyles of the femur (thigh bone). Therefore the gastrocnemius enables both plantarflexion and flexion about the knee (Gray 1918; Saladin 2001; Seeley et al. 2003; Marieb and Hoehn 2013).

Table 2.1 Characteristics of primary ankle-foot complex musculature (Winter 1990)

Muscle	Physiological cross-sectional area (percent across ankle)	Pennation angle
Soleus	41	30
Gastrocnemius	22	15
Tibialis anterior	5	5

The gastrocnemius represents a multijoint muscle, which is capable of contributing torque to more than one joint, such as the knee joint and ankle joint. The mechanical advantage of a specific muscle is uniquely defined according to its origin and insertion. The morphology and spatial representation of a muscle determines the moment arm, which is the displacement between the line normal to the muscle and joint center. Moment arm and muscle force generation derive torque produced about the joint. Notably moment arm varies as a function of joint angle (Winter 1990).

Note the increasing complexity of addressing the encompassing anatomy supporting gait. Muscle physiology and modeling constitutes the actuators enabling gait. Their complexity transcends the role of skeletal structure, which provides structure. However, the ultimate biological system that supports gait in terms of feedback, synchronicity, and modulation is the neurological foundation of gait.

2.4 Neurology of the Ankle-Foot Complex

An entire book of substantial thoroughness may only provide a broad stroke for the substantial influence of neurology regarding gait. As the scope of this topic spans only part of a chapter, the objective is to provide the reader with a general comprehension of the significance of the contribution of neurology in terms of regulating the control of gait from the perspective of advancing transtibial prosthetic technology.

An observant engineer wanting to develop a transtibial prosthesis may consider the neurological command structure that is the foundation for highly specified and preplanned upper limb movement to be representative of the tendencies of the highly synchronous and rhythmic feature of gait. In general such as observation necessitates further refinement. Notably people walk with little allocation of their mental faculties (Watson et al. 2010). A general perspective on the foundational neurology of gait elucidates its considerable contribution to robust and sustainable locomotion.

The supporting neurological foundation for gait is inherently hierarchical in principle. It is derived from cortical, interneuronal, and subcortical aspects. The neurological basis of gait is a synthesis of motor control, sensory feedback, and cognitive input (Dobkin 2003; Kandel et al. 2000; LeMoyne et al. 2008; Watson et al. 2010).

Although locomotion is organized through the central nervous system, it is significantly refined through proprioceptive feedback. Proprioception signifies the body's spatial representation through afferent sensory perception. A broadly accepted concept for regulating locomotion through proprioception is the central pattern generator. A network of interneuronal circuitry characterizes the central pattern generator. The circuitry enables a rhythmic efferent activity that essentially constitutes a self-sustaining motor strategy (Dietz 2002; LeMoyne et al. 2008; Watson et al. 2010).

The monosynaptic reflex represents a highly researched topic of proprioceptive feedback (Dietz 2002; LeMoyne 2010; LeMoyne et al. 2011). The reflex facilitates terrain adaptation (Dietz et al. 1987). Notably the tendon reflex is modulated by contextual supraspinal input. However, the reflex circuitry integrates this input at the spinal cord level and subsequently returns efferent response signal in a manner that is considerably temporally responsive relative to direct cortical motor control (LeMoyne 2010; LeMoyne et al. 2011). For example, the sudden activation of the stretch reflex for the leg extensor musculature could be resultant from a sudden decrement to associated muscle tone (Diamond et al. 1985; LeMoyne 2010; LeMoyne et al. 2011).

The muscle spindle afferent and Golgi tendon organ are foundational sensory components to proprioceptive experience (LeMoyne et al. 2011). The muscle spindle constitutes the primary afferent representation that is the basis for the tendon reflex. The signal derived from the muscle spindle is based on the state of muscle length (Nolte and Sundsten 2002). The muscle spindle is oriented parallel relative to the muscle fibers (Clark et al. 2008). It can measure muscle length in both the context of muscle length and muscle length rate of change (Kandel et al. 2000; Nolte and Sundsten 2002; LeMoyne 2010; LeMoyne et al. 2011).

The other sensory mechanism that provides proprioceptive afferent signal is the Golgi tendon organ. The Golgi tendon organ is oriented in series relative to musculature and tendon. It is activated as a function of muscle tension (Enoka 1988). Its stimulation supports inhibitory features toward efferent motor activation to the contrary effect of the muscle spindle (Nolte and Sundsten 2002; LeMoyne 2010; LeMoyne et al. 2011).

In summary these afferent systems constitute a significant role for the motor learning plasticity of locomotion (LeMoyne et al. 2008). Intuitively the amputation of the entire ankle-foot complex would considerably impair the neurological foundation of gait. For example the terrain adaptation capability of the Achilles tendon reflex would be removed for the residual limb. The residual limb's proprioceptive input to the central pattern generator would be substantially decremented.

The supporting foundations of gait from an anatomical perspective are derived from a considerable level of complexity. From a biomechanical perspective gait is characterized as highly rhythmic with smooth transition (Dobkin 2003; LeMoyne et al. 2008). In order to best define gait cycle, it may be discretized into segmented aspects, such as representative phases and subphases.

2.5 Gait Phases and Subphases

The synchronous and repetitive features of gait are characterized by the alternating activities of each leg while walking. One leg functions as a source of support as the other leg advances and subsequently becomes the base of stability. The gait cycle is characterized as a complete set of gait function. There is no absolute initial aspect for the gait cycle. However, in generic terms the initial contact of the foot striking the floor signifies the commencement of a gait cycle. The gait cycle can also be defined as a stride, which can be represented by a leg making initial contact to the next initial contact of the same leg (Perry 1992).

A gait cycle can be subdivided into two segments defined as stance and swing. Swing phase involves a leg proceeding above ground for preparation of a subsequent stance phase. Stance phase of gait occurs for the duration that the foot is in contact with the ground. There are three readily observable components of stance phase: initial double stance, single stance, and terminal double stance. These features are based on the leg in stance phase and the other leg that is transitioning to swing phase (Perry 1992).

Initial double stance involves the initial contact of one leg in stance phase, while the other leg is transitioning to swing phase. Note that the ground reaction force (load bearing) is generally not equivalent. The next event involves single stance, for which ground contact is sustained by one leg while the other leg advances in swing phase. The final aspect of the perspective of stance phase is expressed as terminal double stance. During this part of stance the opposing leg commences initial contact and the leg of interest finishes stance with toe-off. Weight distribution also is frequently asymmetrical (Perry 1992).

Since gait cycle is characteristically rhythmic, it can be temporally approximated according to stance phase and swing phase. The precise temporal features are unique to the individual. The time duration of each phase is inversely correlated to walking speed. Generally stance phase consists of 60 % and swing phase represents 40 % of the gait cycle. A more specific temporal distribution of the phases of gait is presented in Table 2.2 (Perry 1992).

As shall be later described in Chaps. 8: 'Transtibial powered prostheses: single and dual actuator configurations' and 9: 'The MIT inspired powered prosthesis leading to the commercialized BiOM powered prosthesis, a precedence in transtibial prosthetic technology' a powered prosthesis for people with transtibial amputation can be designed for accommodating either or both aspects of the stance phase and swing phase. From the observational perspective of a person desiring to develop a powered prosthesis, the dorsiflexion for swing phase and stance initiation may signify an important design feature. To a prosthetic designer new to the field of gait analysis, the stance phase may appear to be merely structural with a potential need for some rendition of shock absorbance upon stance initiation. Such a perspective may have led toward the research and development that yielded the Solid Ankle Cushioned Heel (SACH) transtibial prosthesis.

Table 2.2 Temporal distribution of gait (Perry 1992)

Gait phase	Percentage of gait phase	
Stance		60
Initial double stance	10	
Single stance	40	
Terminal double stance	10	
Swing		40

As alluded to regarding the many intricacies of the anatomy supporting the ankle-foot complex, its role is far more than structural. During stance phase a considerable degree of modulation in terms of eccentric and concentric contraction occurs that substantially influences the quality of gait. In fact a considerable majority of mechanical energy is imparted to the gait cycle during stance phase (LeMoyne 2015). Because of this observation, a further functional consideration of the aspects of stance phase is highly warranted.

With regards to various transtibial prostheses, the phases and subphases of gait are contextually relevant to the design objectives of the prosthesis. For the conventional SACH prosthesis, gait may be reduced to the basic stance and swing phases of gait. For more complex prosthetic applications the subphases that comprise the aspects of stance may be contextually unique to the device.

For example the iWalk BiOM enables actuator derived powered plantar flexion about the terminal stance phase. This system requires the identification of controlled plantar flexion, controlled dorsiflexion, and powered plantar flexion subphases of stance (LeMoyne 2015). However, some powered prosthetic applications, such as the PANTOE 1, advocate a segmented foot scenario, which also addresses the heel-off and toe-off components of terminal stance phase (Zhu et al. 2010). For simplicity, the phases and subphases of gait shall be addressed from the perspective of a single component prosthetic foot with actuator powered imparted about the ankle joint.

Gait rhythmically varies from stance to swing phase. During stance the heel establishes initial contact with the ground. Stance phase of gait is a topic of considerable interest respective of current powered prostheses, as actuator power is imparted during this phase. Three aspects of stance are controlled plantar flexion, controlled dorsiflexion, and powered plantar flexion. Stance constitutes approximately 60 % of the gait cycle (Perry 1992; Au et al. 2007a; Au 2007; Fey et al. 2011; LeMoyne 2015).

During the controlled plantar flexion the mechanical representation of the ankle-foot complex can be exemplified through a spring with variable stiffness (Au et al. 2007a, b; Au 2007; Fey et al. 2011; LeMoyne 2015). The anterior tibialis musculature enables eccentric contraction mitigating foot slap, which may lead to long-term degenerative morbidities, while enabling smooth ground contact (Dobkin 2003; Au et al. 2007a, b; LeMoyne et al. 2008; Fey et al. 2011; LeMoyne 2015).

Following controlled plantar flexion is controlled dorsiflexion, which is also representative of a variable stiffness spring. This subphase of stance facilitates energy storage. The energy is released during the next phase powered plantar flexion (Palmer 2002; Au et al. 2006, 2007a, b; Au 2007; Fey et al. 2011; LeMoyne 2015).

Powered plantar flexion entails the release and generation of significant energy about the gait cycle. The concentric activation of the soleus and gastrocnemius plantar flexor muscles imparts substantial torque about the ankle-foot complex (Winter 1983; Dobkin 2003; Au et al. 2006, 2007a, b; Au 2007; Endo et al. 2009; LeMoyne 2015). The gastrocnemius is also a bi-articular muscle. This characteristic enables it to also generate torque about the knee joint, which serves a role in the preparation of transition to swing phase (Winter 1990; Endo et al. 2009).

In fact a major discovery elucidating the significance of plantar flexor musculature was realized during the 1980s in proximity to the timeframe of the rising role of energy storage return prostheses (LeMoyne 2015). Winter found that approximately 80 % of the mechanical power imparted in the gait cycle is resultant from plantar flexor musculature, which occurs during stance phase (Winter 1983; Winter and Sienko 1988; Sanderson and Martin 1997; Dobkin 2003). Certainly over the past three to four decades the contribution and role of stance phase has been far more specified and refined as opposed to the previous centuries of prosthetic applications that merely signify stance phase of gait as structural in significance (LeMoyne 2015).

The remaining 40 % of gait cycle involves the swing phase, for which the leg advances while clearing above ground (Perry 1992). This phase involves a reset of the ankle position for the pending initiation of stance (Au et al. 2007a). Sufficient ankle orientation is extremely important for toe clearance during swing. Circumduction is a compensatory mechanism that can evolve in to an adverse gait pattern in light of chronic inappropriate orientation of the ankle causing toe drag about swing (Dobkin 2003; LeMoyne et al. 2008). With regards to the context specific delineations of gait, the Ossur Proprio Foot is designed to enable clearance of the ankle-foot complex during swing (Ossur).

Conclusion

In order to be capable of developing an authentically biomimetic powered prosthesis an engineering/scientist research and development team should at minimal have a fundamental understanding of the role and contribution of the ankle-foot complex to gait. Covering the knowledge base of this subject comprises multiple fields of biomedical expertise. From an anatomy and physiology perspective the topics of skeletal, muscular, and neurological are concisely summarized. The skeletal features enable both structural and energy absorbing capability. Musculature facilitates both concentric contraction and eccentric contraction for providing acceleration and deceleration qualities about the respective joint. The supporting and associated neurology about the ankle-foot complex empowers the characteristically fluid and synchronous nature of gait. Afferent and efferent pathways contribute to more complex structures, such as the central pattern generator. Afferent representation involves

(continued)

proprioception, known as the body's spatial representation, which applies sensory mechanisms, such as muscle spindle afferents and Golgi tendon organs. With the summary of the foundations of the ankle-foot complex defined, a summary of the rhythmic and synchronous attributes of the gait cycle is covered. Gait can be divided into phases of stance and swing. A successful powered prosthesis design should provide sufficient dorsiflexion about the prosthetic ankle joint for toe clearance. Stance is of particular significance to the domain of powered prosthesis development, and it can be further subdivided into controlled plantar flexion, controlled dorsiflexion, and powered plantar flexion. During the terminal aspect of stance known as powered plantar flexion, a considerable amount of mechanical power is contributed to the gait cycle. Further coverage of the topics discussed in the present chapter can easily span the subject matter of multiple biomedical related books or even the lifetime of a professional biomedical themed career.

References

APMA. www.apma.org

Au SK (2007) Powered ankle-foot prosthesis for the improvement of amputee walking economy. Ph.D. dissertation, MIT, Department of Mechanical Engineering, Cambridge

Au SK, Herr HM (2008) Powered ankle-foot prosthesis. IEEE Robot Autom Mag 15:52–59

Au SK, Dilworth P, Herr H (2006) An ankle-foot emulation system for the study of human walking biomechanics. Proceedings of IEEE international conference on robotics and automation, Orlando, pp 2939–2945

Au SK, Herr H, Weber J, Martinez-Villalpando EC (2007a) Powered ankle-foot prosthesis for the improvement of amputee ambulation. Proceedings of 29th annual international conference IEEE EMBS, Lyon, pp 3020–3026

Au SK, Weber J, Herr H (2007b) Biomechanical design of a powered ankle-foot prosthesis. Proceedings of IEEE 10th international conference rehabilitation robotics, Noordwijk, pp 298–303

Bekey GA (2005) Autonomous robots: from biological inspiration to implementation and control. MIT Press, Cambridge

Burke MJ, Roman V, Wright V (1978) Bone and joint changes in lower limb amputees. Ann Rheum Dis 37:252–254

Clark MA, Lucett SC, Corn RJ (2008) NASM essentials of personal fitness training. Lippincott Williams & Wilkins, Philadelphia

Diamond MC, Scheibel AB, Elson LM (1985) The human brain coloring book. Harper Perennial, New York

Dietz V (2002) Proprioception and locomotor disorders. Nat Rev Neurosci 3:781–790

Dietz V, Quintern J, Sillem M (1987) Stumbling reactions in man: significance of proprioceptive and pre-programmed mechanisms. J Physiol 386:149–163

Dobkin BH (2003) The clinical science of neurologic rehabilitation. Oxford University Press, New York

Endo K, Swart E, Herr H (2009) An artificial gastrocnemius for a transtibial prosthesis. Proceedings of 31st annual international conference IEEE EMBS, Minneapolis, pp 5034–5037

Enoka RM (1988) Neuromechanical basis of kinesiology. Human Kinetics Books, Champaign

Fey NP, Klute GK, Neptune RR (2011) The influence of energy storage and return foot stiffness on walking mechanics and muscle activity in below-knee amputees. Clin Biomech 26:1025–1032

Gray H (1918) Anatomy of the human body. Lea & Febiger, Philadelphia
Hernigou P (2013) Ambroise Paré IV: the early history of artificial limbs (from robotic to prostheses). Int Orthop 37:1195–1197
Hill AV (1938) The heat of shortening and the dynamic constants of muscle. Proc R Soc London B Biol Sci 126:136–195
Huxley H, Hanson J (1954) Changes in the cross-striations of muscle during contraction and stretch and their structural interpretation. Nature 173:973–976
Huxley AF, Niedergerke R (1954) Structural changes in muscle during contraction; interference microscopy of living muscle fibers. Nature 173:971–973
Kandel ER, Schwartz JH, Jessell TM (2000) Principles of neural science. McGraw-Hill, New York
Ker RF, Bennett MB, Bibby SR, Kester RC, Alexander RM (1987) The spring in the arch of the human foot. Nature 325:147–149
LeMoyne R (2010) Wireless quantified reflex device. Ph.D. dissertation, UCLA, Biomedical Engineering IDP, Los Angeles
LeMoyne R (2015) Advances regarding powered prosthesis for transtibial amputation. J Mech Med Biol 15:1–34
LeMoyne R, Coroian C, Mastroianni T, Grundfest W (2008) Virtual proprioception. J Mech Med Biol 8:317–338
LeMoyne R, Mastroianni T, Coroian C, Grundfest W (2011) Tendon reflex and strategies for quantification, with novel methods incorporating wireless accelerometer reflex quantification devices, a perspective review. J Mech Med Biol 11:471–513
Marieb EN, Hoehn K (2013) Human anatomy & physiology. Pearson, New York
Maruyama K (1976) Connectin, an elastic protein from myofibrils. J Biochem 80:405–407
May BJ, Lockard MA (2011) Prosthetics & orthotics in clinical practice: a case study approach. FA Davis, Philadelphia
Morgenroth DC, Segal AD, Zelik KE, Czerniecki JM, Klute GK, Adamczyk PG, Orendurff MS, Hahn ME, Collins SH, Kuo AD (2011) The effect of prosthetic foot push-off on mechanical loading associated with knee osteoarthritis in lower extremity amputees. Gait Posture 34:502–507
Morgenroth DC, Gellhorn AC, Suri P (2012) Osteoarthritis in the disabled population: a mechanical perspective. PM R 4:S20–S27
Mündermann A, Dyrby CO, Andriacchi TP (2005) Secondary gait changes in patients with medial compartment knee osteoarthritis: increased load at the ankle, knee, and hip during walking. Arthritis Rheum 52:2835–2844
Nishikawa KC, Monroy JA, Uyeno TE, Yeo SH, Pai DK, Lindstedt SL (2012) Is titin a 'winding filament'? A new twist on muscle contraction. Proc Biol Sci 279:981–990
Nishikawa KC, Monroy JA, Powers KL, Gilmore LA, Uyeno TA, Lindstedt SL (2013) A molecular basis for intrinsic muscle properties: implications for motor control, chap 6. In: Richardson MJ, Riley MA, Shockley K (eds) Progress in motor control. Springer, New York
Nolan L, Wit A, Dudziñski K, Lees A, Lake M, Wychowañski M (2003) Adjustments in gait symmetry with walking speed in trans-femoral and trans-tibial amputees. Gait Posture 17:142–151
Nolte J, Sundsten JW (2002) The human brain: an introduction to its functional anatomy. Mosby, St. Louis
Opensim. http://opensim.stanford.edu
Ossur. http://www.ossur.com
Palmer ML (2002) Sagittal plane characterization of normal human ankle function across a range of walking gait speeds. Masters of Science Thesis, MIT, Department of Mechanical Engineering, Cambridge
Perry J (1992) Gait analysis: normal and pathological function. Slack, Thorofare
Saladin KS (2001) Anatomy & physiology: the unity of form and function. McGraw-Hill, New York

Sanderson DJ, Martin PE (1997) Lower extremity kinematic and kinetic adaptations in unilateral below-knee amputees during walking. Gait Posture 6:126–136
Seeley RR, Stephens TD, Tate P (2003) Anatomy & physiology. McGraw-Hill, New York
Tester J, Yeo SH, Pai D, Nishikawa K (2012) A new muscle model with implications for actuation and control. Proceedings of 7th annual dynamic walking Conference, Pensacola Beach, pp 1–3
Thelen DG (2003) Adjustment of muscle mechanics model parameters to simulate dynamic contractions in older adults. J Biomech Eng 125:70–77
Thurston AJ (2007) Paré and prosthetics: the early history of artificial limbs. ANZ J Surg 77:1114–1119
Wang K, McClure J, Tu A (1979) Titin: major myofibrillar components of striated muscle. Proc Natl Acad Sci U S A 76:3698–3702
Watson C, Kirkcaldie M, Paxinos G (2010) The brain: an introduction to functional neuroanatomy. Academic Press, New York
Wilson AB Jr (1963) Prosthetics and orthotics research in the United States. Orthop Prosthet Appl J 17:152–160
Winter DA (1983) Energy generation and absorption at the ankle and knee during fast, natural, and slow cadences. Clin Orthop Relat Res 175:147–154
Winter DA (1990) Biomechanics and motor control of human movement. Wiley-Interscience, New York
Winter DA, Sienko SE (1988) Biomechanics of below-knee amputee gait. J Biomech 21:361–367
Yeo SH (2012) Computational modeling of neuromusculoskeletal systems: from filaments to behavior. Ph.D. dissertation, University of British Columbia (Vancouver), Department of Computer Science, Vancouver
Zajac FE (1989) Muscle and tendon: properties, models, scaling, and application to biomechanics and motor control. Crit Rev Biomed Eng 17:359–411
Zhu J, Wang Q, Wang L (2010) PANTOE 1: biomechanical design of powered ankle-foot prosthesis with compliant joints and segmented foot. In Proceedings of IEEE/ASME international conference advanced intelligent mechatronics (AIM), Montréal, pp 31–36

Chapter 3
Prosthetic Gait Asymmetry and Discomfort While Walking with a Transtibial Prosthesis

Abstract In light of the functional disparities of the intact leg relative to a residual leg with a prosthesis asymmetries of the gait cycle can develop. A primary decrement to the residual limb with a prosthesis is the inability to generate powered plantar flexion during the stance phase of gait. Asymmetries in the context of ground reaction force profiles have been demonstrated. Compensatory mechanisms for the can arise, such as amplified work produced about the hip joint of the residual limb. These non-optimal gait patterns can lead to the development of chronic degenerative morbidities, such as osteoporosis, osteoarthritis, scoliosis, and atrophy. People with transtibial amputation can experience amplified metabolic cost during gait, which can lead to reduced optimal gait speed. Another source of discomfort involves the quality of the interface between the socket and the residual limb. Displacement between the socket and residual limb is known as pistoning. These subjects of gait asymmetry and discomfort warrant attention for the development of high quality prosthetic systems.

Keywords Gait asymmetry • Compensatory mechanisms • Ground reaction force • External adduction moment • Pistoning

3.1 Introduction

The previous Chap. 2: 'Ankle-foot complex and the fundamental aspects of gait' clearly establishes the intricacy of the ankle-foot complex and its role with locomotion. The supporting anatomical structures enable considerable adaptation and even reflexivity to the continually changing gait cycle. Clearly a state of the art transtibial prosthesis should facilitate its user with far more than merely structural support.

The majority of transtibial prosthetic devices are less adaptive than the associated intact leg for a person with unilateral amputation. The implication of this situation is the development of gait asymmetry and related compensatory strategies. Since gait is a highly repetitive aspect of an active lifestyle, chronic morbidities, such as joint arthritis and bone degeneration can develop. Reduced energy imparted to the gait cycle can result in amplified metabolic cost while walking (LeMoyne 2015). Another topic of discomfort while walking with a transtibial prosthesis is the

R. LeMoyne, *Advances for Prosthetic Technology*,
DOI 10.1007/978-4-431-55816-3_3

topic of pistoning about the prosthetic interface to the residual limb (Michael 2004; Gholizadeh et al. 2012). The objective of this chapter is to elucidate the nature of prosthetic gait asymmetries, compensatory mechanisms that can arise due to adaptation, chronic morbidities that derive as a consequence, and sources of discomfort, such as increased metabolic cost and pistoning.

3.2 Asymmetry of Gait

A transtibial amputation eliminates considerable functionality of the ankle-foot complex, especially during the stance phase of the gait cycle. The ankle-foot complex facilitates two major roles during the preliminary and terminal aspects of the stance phase of gait. The capacity to control the forward motion of the leg during the initial aspects of gait are regulated by eccentric contraction about the musculature of the ankle joint. Concentric contraction of the plantar flexors provides considerable mechanical power (Winter 1983; Winter and Sienko 1988; Dobkin 2003; LeMoyne et al. 2008; LeMoyne 2015).

The elimination of musculature about the ankle-foot complex from transtibial amputation represents significant challenge for a person with amputation to adapt to such a constrained gait environment, especially with powered plantar flexion removed from the gait cycle (Sanderson and Martin 1997). During the 1980s Winter made a significant research finding that roughly 80 % of the mechanical power contributed to the gait cycle occurs from plantar flexor musculature (Winter 1983; Winter and Sienko 1988; Sanderson and Martin 1997; Dobkin 2003). In tandem with providing significant mechanical power, the plantar flexors provide regulation of the respective leg's forward rotation (Winter 1983; Winter and Sienko 1988). Primary functions of the stance phase of gait are enabling initiation of swing phase, support of body weight, and facilitating the mechanical power of forward propulsion (Sanderson and Martin 1997). Intuitively, in order for a person with an amputation to mimic typical gait activities, disparate motor strategies for the intact leg and residual leg are developed (Sanderson and Martin 1997; LeMoyne 2015).

As a result of the elimination of this significant source of mechanical power, compensatory mechanisms arise. These mechanisms derive from an attempt to offset this deficit of mechanical actuation. For example, a person with an amputation could develop a compensatory strategy by modifying the activity patterns of the residual hip and knee joint. With the notable modification that transtibial amputation induces on anthropometrics and the neural system adaptations develop, particularly with regards to the decrement in motor control (Winter and Sienko 1988). However, as these schemes and their characteristic asymmetry are inherently unnatural, they will likely produce chronic and degenerative morbidities throughout the long term of the recovery and rehabilitation process (Nolan et al. 2003).

Sanderson and Martin applied an experimental study to compare kinematic and kinetic parameters between a set of people with amputation at the transtibial level relative to a group of people without amputation. A passive prosthesis (Flex-Foot) with the ability to store and release energy was applied in the experiment. Data was collected for the intact and residual leg for the person with amputation, and a single limb for the non-amputee (Sanderson and Martin 1997).

Kinematic and kinetic data were acquired through the synchronized use of a force plate and motion capture through video recording. Five anatomical positions were mounted with reflective tape for video analysis: the 5th metatarsal, heel, lateral malleolus, lateral condyle of the knee, and greater trochanter. A video analysis system was incorporated to digitize the kinematic data. The subject was tasked to walk across a walkway at two speeds, which were measured by photocells positioned in a manner to determine speed about the force plate (Sanderson and Martin 1997).

The findings imply that people with amputation apply different motor strategies for the intact limb and residual limb, presumably due to the diminished capacity to provide propulsive force from the residual limb with a passive prosthesis. For the aspects of late stance and early swing the residual limb with the prosthesis demonstrated quantified disparity relative to the non-amputee leg and the intact leg in terms of angular displacement and angular velocity respective of the ankle joint. An inability to modulate propulsive force was discovered. The prosthetic limb did not notably increase for ground reaction force second peak with increasing walking speed, as opposed to the intact limb and non-amputee limb, which demonstrated a proportional relationship (Sanderson and Martin 1997). The second peak of the ground reaction force is correlated with powered plantar flexion at the terminal phase of stance (Winter 1983).

As elucidated in the previous Chap. 2: 'Ankle-foot complex and the fundamental aspects of gait' the ankle-foot complex with its afferent and efferent pathways is capable of adapting to an assortment of self-determined walking scenarios, such as gait speed. Intuitively, a person with transtibial amputation must develop unique compensatory strategies, in order to effectively regulate gait speed. Nolan et al. explored the effect of modulating gait speed on people with transtibial amputation (Nolan et al. 2003).

The investigation focused on subjects with high activity levels, and their basis for unilateral amputation was due to trauma. The subjects with unilateral transtibial amputation all utilized SACH type prostheses. Temporal and kinetic parameters were acquired through an array of eight force sensors positioned in the shoe. The sensors integrated into the shoe were connected to a data logger through a cable mounted about the subject's waist. This experimental environment enabled the subject to walk freely, with minimal constraints (Nolan et al. 2003).

The superposition of all shoe mounted forces sensors resembles the standard force profile produced by a platform mounted force plate. The study elucidated that intact limb of transtibial amputees generates an amplified ground reaction force profile respective of the first peak relative to their prosthetic limb. The asymmetry (intact limb relative to prosthetic limb) of the first peak of ground reaction force increased in proportion with walking speed. The first peak of ground reaction force profile represents the maximal weight acceptance of stance phase. Temporal findings of the study imply that people with amputation reduce swing phase time asymmetrically for the objective of making more symmetrical step times (Nolan et al. 2003). Asymmetric gait patterns with amplified loading about the intact limb for people with amputation have been proposed as a basis for degenerative trends in weight bearing joints (Burke et al. 1978; Nolan et al. 2003).

Silverman et al. investigated the role of compensatory mechanisms in light of various steady state walking velocity scenarios. Subjects participated in the study with their own personal prosthesis, either solid ankle cushioned heel or energy storage and return, which are both passive type prostheses. A more advanced comprehension of compensatory mechanisms was envisioned through analysis of ground reaction force profiles and joint kinetics (Silverman et al. 2008).

In order to quantify the data gait analysis was applied, such as a force plate to measure kinetic data and motion capture system to quantify kinematic data. The motion capture system was represented by eight cameras that measured the bilateral activity through reflective markers of the metatarsal head (first, second, and fifth), heel, dorsal foot, medial malleolus, lateral malleolus, femoral condyles (lateral and medial), greater trochanter, superior iliac spine (anterior and posterior), iliac crest, shoulder, and C-7 vertebrae. The force plate was embedded in a 10 m gait platform. Joint power was the product of joint moment and angular velocity. Joint work was the integral of joint power (Silverman et al. 2008).

The most notable compensatory mechanism involved an increase in positive work for the hip joint of the residual limb. Silverman et al. interpret their findings to imply that amplified residual limb hip extensor activity as a mechanism to regulate greater increase in ground reaction force asymmetry. Future endeavors envision evaluating multiple compensatory strategies for the objective of determining which method best ameliorates adverse joint loading. Also residual limb hip extensor strengthening techniques may protract degenerative joint issues for the intact leg by diminishing dependence (Silverman et al. 2008).

Adamczyk and Kuo further advance the knowledge base of gait asymmetry, as they note that there is no recognized explanation as to why unilateral amputation of the ankle-foot complex leads to asymmetry. They propose a mechanistic examination of the fundamental properties from transtibial amputation and associated compensatory mechanisms that lead to gait asymmetry. Noted is the casual link to loss of power contribution to the gait cycle and the motivation to compensate through other joints providing amplified levels of work. In particular, in consideration of the myriad of compensatory strategies for people with amputation, and individualized and most economical compensatory technique would be subject optimal (Adamczyk and Kuo 2015).

Adamczyk and Kuo created a dynamic walking model for forecasting the influence of unilateral impairment regarding push-off for gait. The model is capable of multiple compensatory strategies when challenged with diminished push-off. The model predicted asymmetries, such as amplified intact limb collision work. In terms of stance phase the intact limb demonstrated slower speed at mid-stance, protracted duration for stance phase, and reduced center of mass velocity relative to the side of the residual (prosthetic) limb. The model implies that positive work about the hip during stance regarding the intact limb. The findings suggest asymmetry of gait is anticipated for persons with unilateral transtibial amputation. Adamczyk and Kuo also note that in consideration of gait economy a degree of asymmetry may be more preferable than endeavoring to develop a more symmetric gait (Adamczyk and Kuo 2015).

3.3 Degenerative and Associated Morbidities from Gait Asymmetry

Gait asymmetry for people with a transtibial prosthesis can induce a considerable array of progressive degeneration and correlated morbidity. The following are some examples:

- Osteoporosis
- Osteoarthritis
- Scoliosis
- Muscle atrophy (LeMoyne 2015)

Osteoporosis involves the reduction in bone tissue mass. This trend makes the respective bone more subject to fracture and more porous (Saladin 2001; Seeley et al. 2003). Osteoporosis has been observed respective of the residual limb (Burke et al. 1978).

Osteoarthritis is characterized by the graduation deterioration of a joint's articular cartilage. This trend can lead to protrusive bone spurs developing into the joint cavity, which impair range of motion and cause discomfort (Saladin 2001; Seeley et al. 2003). Osteoarthritis can develop with the intact knee joint (Burke et al. 1978; Mündermann et al. 2005; Morgenroth et al. 2011).

Scoliosis is another observed feature for people with lower limb amputation (Burke et al. 1978). Scoliosis involves an abnormal curvature about the spinal column. This abnormal curvature encompasses lateral derivation with irregular bending to the side (Saladin 2001; Seeley et al. 2003).

Patterns of muscle atrophy are observed respective of the residual leg relative to the intact leg musculature (Schmalz et al. 2001). Muscle atrophy pertains the reduction in muscle tissue mass due to reduced usage. Distinctive muscle fibers reduce in bulk with ongoing loss of myofibrils (Saladin 2001; Seeley et al. 2003).

Muscle activation changes have been observed to modify muscle characteristics for people with amputation (Winter and Sienko 1988; Schmalz et al. 2001; LeMoyne 2015). Ventral muscles for the upper leg are denoted as the rectus femoris, vastus medialis, vastus intemedialis, vastus lateralis, and sartorius. Dorsal muscles are represented by the gracilis, semitendinosus, and biceps femoris. Ventral musculature of the residual leg demonstrates a considerable degree of atrophy. However, the respective dorsal muscles are comparably unchanged (Schmalz et al. 2001). By contrast the residual limb's flexor (dorsal) muscles display EMG measurements that are relatively hyperactive (Winter and Sienko 1988; Schmalz et al. 2001).

The prosthesis of the residual limb intuitively has substantially reduced powered plantar flexion. This observation associates with an amplified first external adduction moment for the knee joint. The progressive development of osteoarthritis respective of the knee joint is an inferred consequence (Mündermann et al. 2005; Morgenroth et al. 2011; LeMoyne 2015).

There are two prevalent aspects regarding the influence to the severity of external adduction moment:

- Magnitude of ground reaction force
- Orientation of the ground reaction force, in particular medial orientation to the center of rotation for the knee about the coronal plane

The knee joint is comprised of a medial tibiofemoral compartment. The loading of this aspect of the knee joint is associated with the external adduction moment of the knee. The knee joint endures a considerable degree of cyclical load, as gait is a highly frequent activity (Morgenroth et al. 2012). Amplified loading about the intact limb is considered a consequence of the passive prostheses' inability to impart mechanical power about the gait cycle during stance (Winter and Sienko 1988; Morgenroth et al. 2012).

3.4 Amplified Metabolic Cost

A reduction in mechanical work contributed to the stance phase of gait as a consequence of the diminished capacity of a prosthesis to provide muscle like actuation has been correlated to the amplified metabolic cost during gait for persons with transtibial amputation (Houdijk et al. 2009). The characteristic relationship between metabolic cost as a function of walking velocity is a U-shaped function, which can be approximated as a quadratic function. This quadratic function consists of a gait velocity optimal with a minimal metabolic cost, which provides an approximation for a person's preferred walking speed (Genin et al. 2008). As a result of reduced energy contributed to the stance phase with a passive prosthesis, people with amputation generally have an optimal gait speed that is reduced relative to people without amputation. Also, the metabolic cost for typical walking for people with transtibial amputation is generally amplified (Waters et al. 1976; Genin et al. 2008; Houdijk et al. 2009; LeMoyne 2015).

3.5 Pistoning

Another source of discomfort for a person with an amputation is referred to as pistoning. Pistoning involves displacement between the residual limb and the socket. Such displacement occurs during limb ambulation, such as during gait. A major task for the suspension system is to mitigate slippage of the residual limb (Michael 2004; Gholizadeh et al. 2012).

Pistoning has been correlated with the quality of a suspension system's fit to the residual limb. Researchers have primarily quantified the attributes of pistoning through conditions involving standing, which is inherently static. However gait is inherently dynamic. Little research has been conducted for the pistoning of the prosthesis during gait (Eshraghi et al. 2012, Gholizadeh et al. 2012).

Gholizadeh et al. conducted a novel study to quantitatively contrast disparate liners applied to people with transtibial amputation. The basis for quantification was provided by a motion capture system with reflective markers about the prosthetic socket. This experimental configuration enabled the displacement of the prosthesis relative to the residual limb to be accurately acquired (Gholizadeh et al. 2012).

Displacement between the prosthesis and residual limb predominates during the swing phase of gait. Subsequent to the swing phase the initial contact, which is the preliminary aspect of stance, demonstrates notable displacement. For this experimental scenario subject Seal-in X5 liner (Ossur) exhibits diminished displacement relative to the Dermo liner (Ossur) (Gholizadeh et al. 2012).

Conclusion

A perspective regarding the presence of gait asymmetry is important for the development of a well-designed transtibial prosthesis. With the lack of the capacity to generate powered plantar flexion to influence the gait cycle compensatory mechanisms arise, such as increased work produced about the hip joint for the residual limb, which can be potentially consequential in the long term. For example, non-optimal gait patterns can induce chronic degenerative morbidities, such as osteoporosis, osteoarthritis, scoliosis, and atrophy. Other sources of discomfort can arise from increased metabolic cost that can reduce optimal gait speed, and pistoning can be caused from slippage respective of the prosthetic interface and the residual limb. Understanding of the long and near term issues affecting the quality of life for people with transtibial amputation is essential for the research and development of advances in applications for transtibial prostheses.

References

Adamczyk PG, Kuo AD (2015) Mechanisms of gait asymmetry due to push-off deficiency in unilateral amputees. IEEE Trans Neural Syst Rehabil Eng 23:776–785

Burke MJ, Roman V, Wright V (1978) Bone and joint changes in lower limb amputees. Ann Rheum Dis 37:252–254
Dobkin BH (2003) The clinical science of neurologic rehabilitation. Oxford University Press, New York
Eshraghi A, Osman NA, Gholizadeh H, Karimi M, Ali S (2012) Pistoning assessment in lower limb prosthetic sockets. Prosthet Orthot Int 36:15–24
Genin JJ, Bastien GJ, Franck B, Detrembleur C, Willems PA (2008) Effect of speed on the energy cost of walking in unilateral traumatic lower limb amputees. Eur J Appl Physiol 103:655–663
Gholizadeh H, Abu Osman NA, Eshraghi A, Ali S, Sævarsson SK, Wan Abas WA, Pirouzi GH (2012) Transtibial prosthetic suspension: less pistoning versus easy donning and doffing. J Rehabil Res Dev 49:1321–1330
Houdijk H, Pollmann E, Groenewold M, Wiggerts H, Polomski W (2009) The energy cost for the step-to-step transition in amputee walking. Gait Posture 30:35–40
LeMoyne R (2015) Advances regarding powered prosthesis for transtibial amputation. J Mech Med Biol 15:1–34
LeMoyne R, Coroian C, Mastroianni T, Grundfest W (2008) Virtual proprioception. J Mech Med Biol 8:317–338
Michael JW (2004) Prosthetic suspensions and components. In: Smith DG, Michael JW, Bowker JH (eds) Atlas of amputations and limb deficiencies: surgical, prosthetic, and rehabilitation principles. American Academy of Orthopaedic Surgeons, Rosemont, pp 409–425
Morgenroth DC, Segal AD, Zelik KE, Czerniecki JM, Klute GK, Adamczyk PG, Orendurff MS, Hahn ME, Collins SH, Kuo AD (2011) The effect of prosthetic foot push-off on mechanical loading associated with knee osteoarthritis in lower extremity amputees. Gait Posture 34:502–507
Morgenroth DC, Gellhorn AC, Suri P (2012) Osteoarthritis in the disabled population: a mechanical perspective. PM R 4:S20–S27
Mündermann A, Dyrby CO, Andriacchi TP (2005) Secondary gait changes in patients with medial compartment knee osteoarthritis: increased load at the ankle, knee, and hip during walking. Arthritis Rheum 52:2835–2844
Nolan L, Wit A, Dudziñski K, Lees A, Lake M, Wychowañski M (2003) Adjustments in gait symmetry with walking speed in trans-femoral and trans-tibial amputees. Gait Posture 17:142–151
Saladin KS (2001) Anatomy & physiology: the unity of form and function. McGraw-Hill, New York
Sanderson DJ, Martin PE (1997) Lower extremity kinematic and kinetic adaptations in unilateral below-knee amputees during walking. Gait Posture 6:126–136
Schmalz T, Blumentritt S, Reimers CD (2001) Selective thigh muscle atrophy in transtibial amputees: an ultrasonographic study. Arch Orthop Trauma Surg 121:307–312
Seeley RR, Stephens TD, Tate P (2003) Anatomy & physiology. McGraw-Hill, New York
Silverman AK, Fey NP, Portillo A, Walden JG, Bosker G, Neptune RR (2008) Compensatory mechanisms in below-knee amputee gait in response to increasing steady-state walking speeds. Gait Posture 28:602–609
Waters RL, Perry J, Antonelli D, Hislop H (1976) Energy cost of walking of amputees: the influence of level of amputation. J Bone Joint Surg Am 58:42–46
Winter DA (1983) Energy generation and absorption at the ankle and knee during fast, natural, and slow cadences. Clin Orthop Relat Res 175:147–154
Winter DA, Sienko SE (1988) Biomechanics of below-knee amputee gait. J Biomech 21:361–367

Chapter 4
Testing and Evaluation Strategies for the Powered Prosthesis, a Global Perspective

Abstract Testing and evaluation strategies are imperative to establish the efficacy of an experimental powered prosthesis. Biomechanical gait analysis applies the synthesis of equipment; such as force plates and optical motion capture, to acquire kinetic and kinematic parameters. These parameters derive joint characteristics, such as work and power, which can be applied to contrast novel prosthetic platforms. Other gait analysis equipment, such as electromyogram and metabolic analyzers, can determine muscle activation patterns and trends respective of metabolic efficiency while walking. New gait analysis devices function as mobile and wireless platforms. The smartphone and portable media devices are equipped with accelerometer and gyroscope sensors that can remotely monitor gait activity. Traditionally statistical significance is applied to establish a scientifically meaningful disparity between disparate sets of data. However, in the recent decade machine learning has been demonstrated to classify and distinguish between aspects of a feature set implying the eventual capacity to diagnose. Foundational to testing and evaluating transtibial prostheses are the prosthetic alignment procedure and acclimation timeframe.

Keywords Biomechanics • Kinematics • Kinetics • Machine learning • Gait analysis

4.1 Introduction

The biomechanics of gait analysis can provide the objective and quantified basis for establishing the efficacy of a transtibial prosthesis system. Biomechanical analysis involves multiple domains, such as kinematics and kinetics. Kinematics involves the observation and measurement of human movement. Kinematics emphasizes the characteristics of movement, but not the forces that constitute the source of movement. Kinetics encompasses the forces that derive these movements and their associated energetics (Winter 1990).

The forces of the kinetic domain are in derived through the application of a series of equations with the features of kinematics, derived anthropometrics, and measured external forces. Anthropometry is the scientific study of the human body for measurements, such as segment mass, moment of inertia, dimensions, and center of mass.

R. LeMoyne, *Advances for Prosthetic Technology*,
DOI 10.1007/978-4-431-55816-3_4

Anthropometry is highly relevant to prosthesis design, since it is highly correlated with the development of human machine interfaces, such as a prosthesis. Kinematic and kinetic data for human gait can be acquired by conventional gait analysis systems, such as a optical motion capture system and ground reaction force plate, which are generally confined to a gait laboratory (Winter 1990; Dobkin 2003; LeMoyne et al. 2008a, b, 2009a; Huston 2009).

Other traditional systems are relevant to the field of gait analysis, such as electromyogram (EMG) and gas analysis systems, for evaluating metabolic cost. The EMG can evaluate the degree of neuromuscular activity both concentric and eccentric contraction. Metabolic cost can be evaluated according to a gas analysis system, which can be contrasted to a baseline control, for a determination of efficiency, such as during gait (Dobkin 2003; LeMoyne et al. 2008a, b, 2009a).

Other novel wearable applications for the realm of gait analysis have been recently developed. Accelerometers and gyroscopes are sensor aspects of an inertial measurement unit. These aspects have been demonstrated for gait analysis in functionally autonomous environments that are beyond the confines of gait analysis laboratories. Smartphones and portable media devices, such as iPhones and iPods, have been demonstrated with experimentation and post-processing locations occurring geographically remote. Recently the iPhone functioning as a wireless accelerometer platform has been demonstrated for quantifying the acceleration waveform of a transtibial prosthesis during gait (LeMoyne et al. 2009a, 2014a; LeMoyne and Mastroianni 2015).

4.2 Kinematics of Gait (General Operation of Motion Capture Cameras)

Optical motion capture can enable the recording of gait kinematics through 2D representation about the sagittal plane. A 3D motion capture system may be advantageous for certain circumstances, but a 2D recording is sufficient for gait analysis. The sagittal plane of a subject's walking represents the predominant features of interest throughout the gait cycle. Winter advocates the placement of four reflective markers to define the relevant joint angles about the ankle-foot complex. Highly sophisticated and expensive optical motion capture technology with associated software can readily and conveniently quantify gait kinematics (Winter 1990). The objective of this section is to enable the capacity to establish these capabilities with minimal resources.

The general hardware aspects for recording gait kinematics require the operation of a motion capture camera that is mounted to a stable tripod frame. The stability provided by the tripod is imperative, especially in consideration of the sensitivity of high-speed motion capture. The external lighting should also satisfy the constraints of high-speed recording.

Quality external lighting is traditionally provided by either tungsten light bulbs or light emitting diodes (LED's). Tungsten light bulbs are generally much brighter than LED's; however, they also are known to generate considerable heat. As a contrast, LED's are commonly cheaper than tungsten bulbs. Lighting requirements are intensified for scenarios that require color recording. More lighting intensity is needed for increased frame rate.

Ambient lighting, such as fluorescent lighting can pulse, should be avoided during a recording session, since standard fluorescent lighting can pulse at a rate of 60 Hz. Outdoor lighting should be avoided, because intensity could suddenly vary, such as from cloud cover. Another consideration for outdoor scenarios is that intensity can vary also as a function of time. For example a morning recording may have significant disparity in lighting intensity relative to a subsequent next day afternoon recording.

The camera system must be equipped with the ability to convey its data to a local computer for post processing. There are two standard methods for data transfer. The camera can be equipped with a USB cable that can directly connect to the computer for data download. Another option involves the use of a memory card, such as the standard SD card, for data transfer. Once the data parcel for a gait analysis is transferred to a computer for post-processing, it can be reviewed for preliminary quality assessment as a .mov or .mp4 file.

Standard options that may be manipulated through the software interface of the motion capture analysis are: frame rate, resolution, and exposure. The frame rate signifies the number of frames recorded per second, which for example can span between 1 and 2000 Hz for a standard motion capture camera. The magnitude of the frame rate is limited as a function of the external lighting. For instance a high frame rate with standard external lighting would implicate darker images for the motion capture sample.

The frame rate magnitude impacts download time and storage. A protracted download time can adversely affect an experiment that requires a large number of trials. Another consideration is the storage of large amounts of data, which can be especially prohibitive for collaborators who desire to remotely interact. Internet media, such as email and even cloud computing shared document resources, may be limited due to the amount of data recorded.

The resolution of the motion capture camera system is the effective rectangular aspect ratio of the recording. A larger area aspect ratio consisting of a greater quantity of pixels entails a larger vision field, which can be particularly advantageous for a gait analysis experiment. The maximum resolution of a camera is a function of its lens. Generally a larger lens is proportional to greater resolution, but a more expensive camera system.

Another adjustable option for motion capture camera system is the exposure. This parameter represents the lens' level of exposure to light. Greater exposure provides more light to the lens, which enables better image contrast.

The optimal tuning of these parameters facilitates the ideal image with crisp definition of the selected markers throughout the gait cycle. The marker selection is critical for proper implementation. For example, white markers should be designated for a color or dark background.

The optical motion capture camera systems enable the acquisition of data for the scope of kinematics. This apparatus can enable the acquisition of the spatial temporal features of the gait cycle with minimal encumbrance. The motion capture system can evaluate the efficacy of an experimental transtibial prosthesis relative to a conventional prosthesis. Another important aspect of the biomechanical analysis of gait is kinetics. The kinetics of gait are readily measured through the application of a ground reaction force system.

4.3 Kinetics of Gait (General Operation of Ground Reaction Force Plate)

The ground reaction force plate is relatively simpler to operate than the motion capture system. A force plate is characteristically stationary and is normally embedded into a walkway platform for a conventional gait analysis laboratory. The force plate generates an electrical signal proportional to the magnitude of force applied, such as by a person in stance phase of gait. Four types of transducers for measuring force involve piezoelectric effect, piezo-resistivity, capacitors, and strain gauges (Winter 1990; Dobkin 2003; LeMoyne et al. 2008b, 2009a).

The derived force vector is three-dimensional in nature. The vertical component of the ground reaction force reveals a distinctive double hump profile. The first maxima represents braking phase of stance, and the second maxima pertains to the push-off aspect of stance. This profile is sufficiently distinct, such that the ground reaction force profile has been successfully applied as a feature set for machine learning classification (Ishikawa et al. 2005; Fey et al. 2011; LeMoyne 2015).

In a conventional gait laboratory the force plate is generally embedded into a platform that is the focal for gait experimentation. Because the force plate is stationary and the subject's starting position is variable, a subject with the assistant of the gait analysis team must determine the correct starting position for the subject based on the locomotive attributes of the subject. Once the correct starting position is ascertained, the subject should commence gait with their neck and line of site oriented in a naturally representative manner.

There are more suggested criteria advised for an experimental protocol that enables the gait analysis to be representative of a subject's natural gait features. A sufficient distance between the starting position and force plate should be established such that the subject may reach steady state walking conditions. In general the subject may be requested to walk at an array of velocity settings, such as slow, medium (self-selected), and fast. The self-selected velocity is according to the subject's discretion. The slow and fast gait velocities may be recognized through a pulse tone, such as a metronome, and confirmed by a stop-watch.

The software operation of the force plate is relatively simple by comparison to the procedures for using the optical motion capture analysis system. In general the force plate may be set to a standard sampling rate, such as 1000 Hz, and upon being activated it should be provided with a warm-up duration for preliminary calibration. A force plate records the force signal for an assigned duration. The force signal recording is activated, terminated, and saved at the discretion of the operator.

The force plate serves a unique role for gait analysis. One of the design objectives of current and future state of the art powered prostheses for subjects with transtibial amputation is to enable the natural stance subphases of controlled plantar flexion, controlled dorsiflexion, and powered plantar flexion that occur during the gait cycle (LeMoyne 2015). The force plate can record and evaluate these features, and then contrast the efficacy of a new prosthesis design relative to natural gait or a conventional prosthesis.

4.4 Other Device for Gait Analysis (EMG and Metabolic Analysis)

Two other traditional gait analysis systems are the EMG and metabolic analysis device. The EMG measures neuromuscular activity (activation) to an assigned muscle group. The signal of an EMG sensor can derive patterns of activation regarding a set of muscles and their associated synchronicity. With this information muscle control can be derived (Dobkin 2003; LeMoyne et al. 2008b, 2009a; LeMoyne 2015).

Generally, the surface electrodes of an EMG system are positioned about the body of the muscle or also multiple points of a targeted muscle. An interface is placed in a standard fashion between the subject's body and muscle surface electrode, such as an electro-cream for adherence and signal transmission. The signal acquisition can be improved by abrading the skin local to the target muscle.

The EMG system consists of five general components. A surface electrode receives the signal conveys it to a wire. The electrode wires, such as California fine wire, transmit the signal. The transmission amplifier's role is to amply the EMG signal to the data translator. The data translator sends the amplified data to a local computer. The local computer is equipped with associated software for processing the EMG signal data.

Metabolic analysis can be provided through a portable gas analysis system. The device measures the consumption of oxygen. This data can be contrasted to a control or resting baseline scenario. The standard transtibial prosthesis lacks the ability to provide the user with the capacity to emulate powered plantar flexion demonstrated by the intact leg. This condition can result in a decremented metabolic efficiency, which can be revealed by metabolic analysis (LeMoyne 2015).

4.5 Synchronization of Gait Analysis System and Signal Processing

Once a gait analysis trial sample has been acquired and stored the data package may need to undergo signal processing. Especially when applying a high sampling rate to a gait analysis experiment that greatly exceeds the frequency content of standard gait characteristics signal processing is highly relevant. For example a disturbance in the 100 Hz frequency range is likely due to the qualities of the gait analysis system, not a subject's natural motion. In this case a low pass filter, such as a 10 Hz low pass Butterworth filter, would be appropriate for the signal processing (Winter 1990).

There is also a limit for the minimal sampling rate of a sensor system also. The minimal sampling threshold can be established based on the Nyquist criterion. The Nyquist criterion defines the minimal sampling frequency as twice the upper threshold of the recorded frequency content (LeMoyne et al. 2009a). For example, Saremi et al. used a sampling rate of 32 Hz for a portable accelerometer system for gait analysis, which implies the anticipated upper threshold of the frequency domain for the gait cycle as 16 Hz (Saremi et al. 2006; LeMoyne et al. 2009a).

The synchronization of multiple gait analysis devices enables the synthesis of their respective signals, such as for the computation of ankle power and ankle work during the stance phase. In order to achieve this objective the motion capture camera and ground reaction force plate must have their signals synchronized. One strategy for synchronizing these signals is through a quantifiable and mutual event, such as initial contact commencing stance phase. The two signals could be synchronized according to a criteria, such as when the time rate of change in vertical displacement about a reflective marker about the heel approaches zero and the normal ground reaction force exceeds a threshold.

Another strategy is to synchronize the two gait analysis system signals according to an extraneous signal that both devices emulate for the objective of mutual synchronization. For example, multiple gait analysis systems could synchronize according to a generated sinusoidal pulse. This alternative is particularly useful for synchronizing and EMG signal to other gait analysis systems.

4.6 Post-processing of Optical Motion Capture Data

Upon acquisition of the motion capture data by reflective marker, the data can be post-processed for the acquisition of joint angles and joint angular rotation rates. Each frame of the data package has a temporal quality for developing spatial-temporal relationships. Identifying a position on the marker develops the spatial-temporal relationship of the marker data set during gait. Multiple marker positions can be used to define angular parameters, such as joint angles and joint angular rotation rates (Winter 1990). The angular data be acquired through video analysis software systems, and some exist as free software packages, such as ImageJ, Kinovea, and Tracker (ImageJ; Kinovea; Tracker).

4.7 Smartphones and Portable Media Devices for Gait Analysis

During 2010 LeMoyne et al. demonstrated the value of applying a smartphone for the context of gait analysis. A sensor package that consists of a three dimensional accelerometer enables the smartphone to record movement status. This capability enables the smartphone to quantify gait status. The smartphone is equipped with a software platform that enables a considerable degree of application versatility (LeMoyne et al. 2010a; LeMoyne and Mastroianni 2015).

A software application enables the smartphone to function as a wireless accelerometer platform. Each gait analysis trial can be recorded and wirelessly conveyed through the Internet as an email attachment. Preliminary testing and evaluation demonstrated a considerable level of accuracy and reliability. The smartphone constitutes a wireless accelerometer node, and it can be mounted about any commonly identified anatomical feature, such as proximal to the knee joint, ankle joint, and lumbar aspect of the spine (LeMoyne et al. 2010a, b, c; LeMoyne and Mastroianni 2015).

During 2011 LeMoyne et al. further evolved the concept of wireless accelerometer platforms to the domain of portable media devices. Portable media devices can potentially operate using the same software platform as the smartphone; therefore they can utilize the same software application. The same software application demonstrated on the smartphone can enable the portable media device to function as a wireless accelerometer platform with wireless transmission of the recording through the Internet as an email package. Portable media devices have also demonstrated a considerable degree of accuracy and reliability for the field of gait analysis (LeMoyne et al. 2011; LeMoyne and Mastroianni 2012, 2015).

The potential for smartphones and portable media devices has been identified as a domain of considerable potential for gait analysis. Performance capabilities of these systems are envisioned to improve dramatically in the near future in terms of software, processing, battery lifetime, mass properties, and sensor package. Future advances envision the use of the gyroscope signal and tandem gyroscope and accelerometer signals for the field of gait analysis (LeMoyne and Mastroianni 2015).

A major advantage of this type of wireless accelerometer platform for gait analysis is the effective autonomy of the device. By contrast to conventional gait analysis devices, the smartphones and portable media devices can be applied at the convenience of a subject's choice, such as a familiar homebound setting. For simplicity, the operation of these devices is anticipated to be feasibly operated by the subject. The experimentation site and post-processing site can be located anywhere in the world with Internet accessibility to email. Simple anatomical mounted positions have been emphasized, with mounting by elastic band, such as a sock (LeMoyne 2015). However, for mounting a smartphone to a prosthetic limb, more contextually robust methods are addressed.

As opposed to using an elastic band for mounting the smartphone to a limb, 3D printing can be incorporated. During 2014 LeMoyne et al. applied a 3D printed adapter interface to mount a smartphone to a passive prosthesis. Rather than using an anatomical mounting procedure, the 3D printed adapter with smartphone was placed at a determined linear displacement about the passive prosthesis. The experimental site and post-processing site were relatively remotely positioned. The smartphone as a wireless accelerometer platform with a 3D printed adapter for gait analysis of a passive prosthesis displays considerable accuracy and reliability (LeMoyne et al. 2014a).

Future evolution of smartphone and portable media devices also envision advances regarding the training of beneficial and optimal motor strategies through feedback (LeMoyne et al. 2008a, 2009a; LeMoyne and Mastroianni 2015). Machine learning may be applied to tandem processing of the accelerometer signal as a feature set. Such a software platform could potentially augment diagnostic acuity of a proposed therapy and rehabilitation strategy.

4.8 The Role of Gait Analysis Systems for Evaluation of Transtibial Prostheses

Currently there are many transtibial prostheses that are the subject of research, development, test, and evaluation. The quantification of relevant gait parameters can establish an objective contrast relative to a current conventional transtibial prosthesis. The role of gait analysis systems is integral toward achieving these objectives (LeMoyne 2015).

Metabolic analysis can evaluate the amount of energy expenditure during a subject's walking. Contrasting the subject to a well-defined baseline can designate the metabolic efficiency. Since people with transtibial amputation lack the ability to generate power about the ankle-foot complex. This characteristic can cause a subject with amputation to have decremented metabolic efficiency relative to comparable people without amputation. Metabolic analysis can in particular evaluate the efficacy of a powered transtibial prosthesis that aims to impart mechanical work about the subphases of stance, such as powered plantar flexion (LeMoyne 2015).

The EMG system can evaluate the activation levels of muscles about the intact limb and residual limb. Intuitively a subject with transtibial amputation may develop compensatory gait patterns that involve off-nominal muscle activation patterns. A novel transtibial prosthesis may be evaluated with EMG sensors to determine if the prosthesis ameliorates these adverse tendencies (LeMoyne 2015).

Optical motion capture and ground reaction force systems can be separately applied or synchronized to quantitatively evaluate the characteristics of a novel prosthesis. The motion capture system alone can determine useful gait parameters, such as minimal foot clearance and range of motion about the ankle. The ground reaction force plate can measure normal force produced by the foot during stance phase and also identify distinct features of stance subphases, such as controlled plantar flexion, controlled dorsiflexion, and powered plantar flexion (LeMoyne 2015).

4.9 Computation of Ankle Power and Work

With the synchronization of the optical motion capture and ground reaction force systems, their parameters can be processed with a series of equations to determine the work and power about the ankle during stance. These derived values are of considerable interest for the design and evaluation of new powered prosthesis applications for transtibial amputation (Winter 1990; LeMoyne 2015).

Seven reflective markers are advocated by Winter to define from a kinematic perspective the spatial orientation of the lower limb. Markers 1 and 2 are positioned on the thigh proximal to the hip joint and knee joint, respectively. Markers 3 and 4 are aligned with the tibia proximal to the knee joint and ankle joint, respectively. Marker 5 is located about the heel (calcaneus). Marker 6 is located at the joint system between the toes and foot (metatarsophalangeal joint). Marker 7 is most distal respective of the toes (distal phalanges). For the following analysis markers 3, 4, 5, and 6 are most relevant (Winter 1990).

Power about the ankle can be derived by the following relation involves moment about the ankle and joint angular velocity:

$$
\begin{aligned}
&P = M\omega \\
&P : Power \\
&M : Moment \\
&\omega : Joint\ angular\ velocity \\
&\omega = \frac{d\theta}{dt} \\
&\theta_{ankle} = \theta_{43} - \theta_{65} + 90 \\
&\theta : Angle
\end{aligned}
$$

(Winter 1990)

Work about the ankle can be derived based on the integration of the power relation by time and between to discrete temporal bounds:

$$W = \int_{t_1}^{t_2} P dt$$

(Winter 1990)

4.10 Derivation of Moment (Torque) About the Ankle

The derivation of moment (torque) about a joint, such as the ankle, consists of the amalgamation of kinetics through a force plate and kinematics through optical motion capture data. The spatial orientation data can be post-processed into angular data.

$$\theta_{ij} = arctan\left(\frac{y_j - y_i}{x_j - x_i}\right)$$
$$i, j : Specified\ marker\ position$$
$$x : x - direction\ orientation$$
$$y : y - direction\ orientation$$
$$\theta_{ij} : Angular\ orientation\ respective\ of\ i\ and\ j\ marker\ position$$

The velocity and acceleration can be derived through their respective derivatives, such that:

$$v = \frac{d(d(t))}{dt},\ a = \frac{dv}{dt}, a = \frac{d^2(d(t))}{dt^2}$$

$$\omega = \frac{d(\theta(t))}{dt},\ \alpha = \frac{d\omega}{dt}, \alpha = \frac{d^2(\theta(t))}{dt^2}$$

A free body diagram is then incorporated to analyze the forces and moments acting upon the joint under consideration, such as the ankle. Mass properties of the foot, center of mass, and moment of inertia can be established through anthropometric data. Each joint respective of the human anatomy functions through the influence of muscle moments, reaction forces, and forces due to gravity (Winter 1990).

With the free body diagram defining the moments and forces about the joint under consideration the equations representing the summation of forces and summation of moments can be applied. First solve the force summation equation, and then solve the moment summation equation:

$$\Sigma F_x = ma_x$$
$$\Sigma F_y = ma_y$$
$$\Sigma F : Summation\ of\ forces$$
$$m : Mass$$
$$a : Acceleration$$
$$x : x - direction\ orientation$$
$$y : y - direction\ orientation$$

Note that y-direction force summation includes the segment mass-gravity term (mg). Solve for moment (torque) about a joint, such as the ankle, based on the moment summation:

$$\Sigma M = I\alpha$$
$$\Sigma M : Summation\ of\ moments$$
$$I : Moment\ of\ inertia$$
$$\alpha : Angular\ acceleration$$

(Winter 1990)

Another strategy for determining joint torque (moment) was developed by Okada et al.:

$$\begin{aligned} M_{az} &= -r_{dx} \cdot F_y + r_{dy} \cdot F_x - r_{px} \cdot (m \cdot a_y - F_y - m \cdot g) + r_{py} \cdot (m \cdot a_x - F_x) + I_z \cdot \alpha_z \\ &= -r_{dx} \cdot F_y + r_{dy} \cdot F_x - r_{px} \cdot m \cdot a_y + r_{px} \cdot F_y + r_{px} \cdot m \cdot g + r_{py} \cdot m \cdot a_x - r_{py} \cdot F_x + I_z \cdot \alpha_z \\ &= (r_{dy} - r_{py}) \cdot F_x + (r_{px} - r_{dx}) \cdot F_y + r_{py} \cdot m \cdot a_x + r_{px} \cdot m \cdot (g - a_y) + I_z \cdot \alpha_z \end{aligned}$$

(Okada et al. 2007)

This approach incorporates a link-segment model using 2D inverse dynamics about the sagittal plane. F_x and F_y are horizontal and vertical ground reaction forces. The mass of the foot is m. Linear accelerations about the foot's center of mass are represented by a_x and a_y. The acceleration of gravity is g. I_z is the principal moment of inertia for the foot about the center of mass. The angular acceleration of the foot is a_z. Position vectors for the point of ground reaction force from the foot center of mass are r_{dx} and r_{dy}. The position vectors for the ankle joint center from the foot center of mass are r_{px} and r_{py} (Okada et al. 2007).

4.11 Derivation of Energy Expenditure as a Function of Metabolic Analysis System

A metabolic analysis system measures the amount of oxygen utilized while breathing. The following function can be applied to determine the energy expenditure as a function of oxygen concentration inhaled/exhaled.

$$E = 21(V \cdot \Delta O_2)$$
$$E : Energy\ Expenditure\ (kJ)$$
$$V : Ventilation\ Rate$$
$$\Delta O_2 : Oxygen\ concentration\ difference\ (inhaled/exhaled)$$

(Brockway 1987; LeMoyne 2015)

4.12 Statistical Significance and Machine Learning Classification for Gait Analysis

Once a control and experimental data set have been synthesized to produce data sets for contrast, it is useful to compare these values for statistical significance. Generally alpha is set to 0.05 for testing for statistical significance of a collection of means. An analysis of variance (ANOVA) is a standard statistical process for determining statistical significance. The ANOVA is a standard statistical approach for comparing means of respective groups for statistical significance (Bland 2000).

Rather than only comparing a set of means for statistical significance, machine learning takes a set of features for a class of data. Based on the feature set machine learning can derive a classification accuracy which can be applied for predictive and ideally diagnostic capabilities. Fundamental examples are the application of machine learning for voice recognition and facial identification (Hall et al. 2009; LeMoyne et al. 2009a; Witten et al. 2011; Weka). The success of machine learning has led toward applications regarding the context of gait analysis.

Within the span of roughly a decade the utility of machine learning has been applied to domain of gait analysis. Begg and Kamruzzaman successfully applied the support vector machine, which is a robust machine learning algorithm, for the objective of classifying on the basis of a feature set derived from minimal foot clearance while walking. The research facilitated the capacity to two perceptibly disparate sets of gait configurations, such as respective of the young and elderly (Begg and Kamruzzaman 2005). Machine learning has been further applied to before and after surgery scenarios. For example, the support vector machine has been applied toward efficaciously classifying subjects that underwent knee surgery respective of their pre-surgery and post-surgery status (Levinger et al. 2007; Levinger et al. 2009). Other machine learning techniques have been applied to gait analysis, such as the artificial neural network. The data signal from an insole pressure pattern demonstrated the capacity to derive ground reaction force data respective of the training range in terms of an intra-subject perspective (Savelberg and de Lange 1999).

As an array of machine learning platforms exist, the preferable machine learning application is contextually specific to the objectives of the research team and the perspective of the experiment. LeMoyne et al. selected logistic regression for distinguishing between feature sets of a subject's affected leg and unaffected leg based on the signal of a force plate. Logistic regression was identified as applying the entire data space to designate full distribution change among the pathology. By contrast, the support vector machine pertains to the development of a delineating hyperplane established with consideration of the most challenging to classify trials (LeMoyne et al. 2014b).

A foundational aspect of conducting appropriate machine learning is the establishment of a proper feature set that appropriately characterizes the experiment and the objectives of the researchers. A suitable feature set for a machine learning algorithm involves a pertinent set of data that best describes an experiment. For example, LeMoyne et al. incorporated a force plate derived feature set that incorporated the local maxima of the brake and push-off phase of stance and their temporal attributes, such as temporal disparity, rise time, and fall time. Using logistic regression to classify between a hemiplegic affected and unaffected limb set, LeMoyne et al. achieve 100 % classification (LeMoyne et al. 2014b).

A standard machine learning platform is the Waikato Environment for Knowledge Analysis (WEKA). This platform is free software offered by the University of Waikato. Some of the available machine learning algorithms that WEKA offers are the decision tree, naïve Bayes, support vector machine, logistic regression, and multilayer perceptron neural network. The attributes for the WEKA machine learning platform are consolidated into a Attribute-Relation File Format (ARFF). The ARFF can be derived from a simple Microsoft Excel Comma-Separated-Value file or an application specific software program that extracts the attributes of a feature set and condenses the results into a text file conforming to the ARFF configuration (Hall et al. 2009; Witten et al. 2011; Weka).

4.13 Machine Learning for Classification of Prosthesis Type

LeMoyne et al. has further expanded the domain of machine learning for the context of prosthetic applications. The scope of the research objective was to utilize machine learning for the role of classifying two disparate classes of transtibial prostheses based on recorded signal of a conventional gait analysis system. Based on the operational simplicity and convenience of setting, a force plate mounted to a gait platform in a gait laboratory was selected. The subject was tasked to traverse the gait platform with the prosthesis contacting the force plate during stance phase. The research comprised the perspective relevant to engineering proof of concept (LeMoyne et al. 2015a).

The goal of the research was to distinguish between two different types of prosthesis Solid Ankle Cushioned Heel (SACH) and an iWalk BiOM powered prosthesis. WEKA provides many machine learning applications for classifying a feature set. A support vector machine was selected given its capacity to delineate a feature set through the application of a support vector (Hall et al. 2009; LeMoyne et al. 2015a).

The derivation of the pertinent feature set is readily established by consideration of the two types of prostheses, which demonstrate considerable functional disparities. The two selected prostheses were the Solid Ankle Cushioned Heel (SACH) and iWalk BiOM powered prosthesis. The SACH was the product of major institutions of the United States of America conducting research and development subsequent to the Second World War (Wilson 1963). The primary role of the SACH is to provide the user with structural support, as the prosthesis is passive in nature (LeMoyne 2015).

On the scale of a quarter of a century later the substantial influence of powered plantar flexion was better comprehended. In response to this major discovery Herr et al. progressively advanced a prostheses capable of generating powered plantar flexion. This type of powered prosthesis better emulated intact gait, while incorporating a series elastic actuator (Herr and Grabowski 2012; LeMoyne 2015).

The loading of the stance phase imparts a unique force signature, which can be recorded by a force plate (Perry 1992; Dobkin 2003; LeMoyne et al. 2008a; LeMoyne 2015). The feature set of the force plate recording can be readily acquired based on distinct characteristics of the force signal (LeMoyne et al. 2015a). Stance initiation entails a notable preliminary maximum upon loading during stance initiation, which is often referred to as braking. The force plate signal then reduces to a local maximum. At the terminal portion of stance the ankle-foot complex provides powered plantar flexion about the gait cycle, which generates another local maxima, which is generally denoted as push off (Ishikawa et al. 2005; Fey et al. 2011; LeMoyne 2015).

With the understanding of the relevance of the force plate profile well established the next task was to reduce the data of the force plate signal to a feature set. LeMoyne et al. applied both temporal parameters and kinetic parameters from the stance phase of gait to populate the feature set. The feature set was synthesized into an Attribute-Relation File Format (ARFF) consisting of six attributes. The ARFF consisted of five numeric attributes, based on the consideration of significant characteristics of the force plate recording. Two temporal parameters were:

- Rise time to brake (first local maximum)
- Fall time from push off (second local maximum) (LeMoyne et al. 2015a)

The initial and final times for the stance force signal were based on the signal exceeding a relative threshold. The feature set incorporated three kinetic parameters:

- Local maximum during brake
- Local maximum during push off
- Mean of the stance force signal (LeMoyne et al. 2015a)

The class attribute pertained to the two types of prosthesis. A SACH without active powered plantar flexion during the terminal aspect of stance represented the passive prosthesis. The iWalk BiOM that contributes powered plantar flexion to the terminal aspect of stance primarily through a series elastic actuator represented the powered prosthesis (LeMoyne et al. 2015a).

With the feature set acquired by means of a force plate signal the support vector machine attained 100 % classification between the SACH passive prosthesis and the iWalk BiOM powered prosthesis. The implications of the findings signify that a feature set derived from a conventional gait analysis platform can be applied to the context of machine learning for classifying disparate types of transtibial prostheses, such as passive prosthesis and powered prosthesis. Further machine learning analysis can be conducted by further segmenting the feature set into specifically a temporal feature set and a kinetic feature set. The implication of conducting this further machine learning analysis is the capacity to further define the most predominant aspects within the feature set (LeMoyne et al. 2015a).

The temporal feature set was comprised of two numeric attributes (the rise time to brake and the fall time from push off). The temporal feature set achieved 100 % classification through the use of the support vector machine, which is a machine learning application provided by WEKA. The kinetic feature set consisted of three numeric attributes based on the force plate profile (the local maximum of force at brake, the local maximum of force at push off, and the average force encompassing the stance force profile). The kinetic feature set achieved 80 % classification based on the support vector machine (LeMoyne et al. 2015a). The implication of this disparity in classification accuracy suggests that the for this subject specific experiment the temporal aspects of the feature set are predominant relative to the kinetic aspects of the feature set (Hall et al. 2009; LeMoyne et al. 2015a).

With the capacity to demonstrate considerable classification accuracy accomplished there are many implications for the role of machine learning for providing a person with a powered prosthesis an optimal software platform. In general a powered prosthesis can intuitively consist of a considerable quantity of tuning parameters. Attaining the optimal tuning could be a trial and error intensive task. Using the telemetry acquired from a powered prosthesis a pertinent feature set could be derived. Machine learning could be applied to enable augmented diagnostic acuity regarding a set of tuning parameters. A future goal is to classify between disparate software platforms. The implications of integrating machine learning into the role of optimizing a powered prosthesis' software platform and tuning parameters may augment to the quality of life and activity levels for people with amputation.

Future endeavors may also entail closed loop feedback between the powered prosthesis and person with amputation. LeMoyne et al. have demonstrated the concept of closed loop feedback for gait during 2008, and the concept was referred to as Virtual Proprioception. Virtual Proprioception encompasses the application of wireless accelerometers for auditory and visual feedback regarding the functional disparity of hemiplegic gait (LeMoyne et al. 2008a, c). Recently in 2015, LeMoyne et al. applied a preliminary closed loop feedback technique for the efficacy of deep brain stimulation using a smartphone as a wireless accelerometer platform, constituting a mechatronic system. The application was capable of distinguishing from an observational perspective and in the context of machine learning a subject's essential tremor with the deep brain stimulator in 'on' and 'off' mode (LeMoyne et al. 2015b, c).

4.14 Subject Inclusion Criteria for an Experimental Design

The inclusion criteria that establishes the subject cohesion has a substantial impact respective of the research implications and findings of a respective gait study. Standard to the majority of gait studies are subject parameters, such as age, height, mass, and gender. However the subject inclusion criteria for people with amputations is considerably more involved and complex. For example a subject's residual limb length can possibly influence their outcome potential regarding a prosthesis research and development study (LeMoyne 2015).

Multiple aspects relevant to the experimental design have been identified. These subjects are briefly summarized with a pending more thorough consideration:

- Nature of amputation
- Duration of years following amputation and type of prosthesis
- Rehabilitation status and associated mobility capability
- Acclimation period to new prosthesis

The proper consideration of the above criteria can likely have considerable influence with regards to the quality of a research study intended to establish the efficacy of a novel prosthetic application (LeMoyne 2015).

A comprehension of nature of a person's amputation can affect the relevance of a prosthetic study. For example, the etiology leading to the amputation may entail other morbidities. A soldier surviving an amputation due to an improvised explosive device may other issues to contend with, such as traumatic brain injury. A subject with neuro-motor impairments, such as traumatic brain injury, may have difficulty adapting to a novel motor control strategy (LeMoyne et al. 2008a, c, 2009b, 2013). Neurological and musculoskeletal disorders can adversely affect the quality of a study (Morgenroth et al. 2011; LeMoyne 2015). A subject inclusion criteria can also down-select people with pulmonary and cardiovascular disorders associated with the etiology of their amputation (Herr and Grabowski 2012; LeMoyne 2015).

Amputations are frequently attributed to trauma. For example, transtibial amputation due to traumatic injuries, such as a motorcycle accident, gunshot, or anti-personnel ordinance, may constrain the nature of the amputation, without complicating factors, such as comorbidities. Subject inclusion criteria can also pertain to whether the subject has experienced a unilateral amputation or a bilateral amputation (Endo et al. 2009; Herr and Grabowski 2012; LeMoyne 2015).

The subject's time to adapt to the new conditions of an amputation and the subject's preferred prosthesis can impact the quality of a prosthetic study (LeMoyne 2015). Inclusion criteria can be refined toward focusing on people who use a prosthesis with passive elasticity (Herr and Grabowski 2012). In general the adaptation time subsequent to an amputation is at the discretion of the research team, however, generally on the order of years (LeMoyne 2015). Houdijk et al. applied a criterion with a minimum one-year for the usage of a prosthesis (Houdijk et al. 2009). Other research teams have expanded their prosthesis usage criteria for longer durations. Herr et al. incorporated a minimal two year threshold regarding post amputation (Herr and Grabowski 2012).

The extent of a person with amputation's rehabilitation progress can have major impact regarding the implications of a prosthesis research and development study. As entailed in Chap. 1: 'Amputations and prostheses, a topic of global concern' the Special Interest Group in Amputee Medicine (SIGAM) incorporates six clinical grades to characterize the mobility capacity of a person with an amputation (Ryall et al. 2003). Mancinelli et al. applied a study that included confirmed highly level ambulators who achieve the threshold spanning from SIGAM level E to F (Mancinelli et al. 2011). Other studies have established a time threshold for which a person with amputation has not required an assistive device (Darter and Wilken 2014).

4.15 Adaptation Time Span for an Experimental Prosthesis

The time span for which a person with an amputation is permitted to acclimate to an experimental prosthesis imparts a critical influence on the efficacy and relevance of the research endeavor. The acclimation duration also impacts budgetary and scheduling constraints. The research team would also need to define if the subject would be permitted to utilize an experimental prosthesis over the span of days, which implies personalized and homebound usage. Such constraints may complicate Institutional Review Board approval. Other alternatives would involve the subject visiting the research site, such as a gait laboratory, and acclimating to the experimental prosthesis under the constraints of a discrete amount of time and a gait laboratory setting. All of these issues must be balanced in consideration of providing optimal experimental impact in consideration of the subject's schedule constraints and the available resources of the research team (LeMoyne 2015).

The significance of the acclimation period is established through the presumption of motor plasticity (Dietz 2002; LeMoyne et al. 2008a; LeMoyne 2015). Afferent feedback, such as spatial representation through proprioception provided significant influence to the synchronous and rhythmic characteristics of human locomotion. With an experimental prosthetic device, such as a powered prosthesis augmenting the powered plantar flexion phase of stance, the user undergoes an adaptation to the new influence to the gait cycle. Compensatory influences may ameliorate with progressive acclimation. The plasticity response to a new motor pattern logically becomes more established with prolonged acclimation (LeMoyne et al. 2008a; LeMoyne 2015).

In consideration of recent prosthetic research endeavors, approximately 43 days were assigned to the acclimation period. This experimental research incorporated the BiOM powered prosthesis, which is considered as the state of the art for powered prostheses. A significantly unique feature of the BiOM powered prosthesis is the ability to provide the user with powered plantar flexion during the terminal aspect of stance phase. Another issue for the basis of warranting about 43 days for acclimation with regards to this experimental research is the application of relatively complex motor tasks, such as ascending a stairway (Aldridge et al. 2012).

In general the budget and time constraints for an experimental study would be adversely affected with such a protracted acclimation timeframe on the order of months. As an alternative to adapting to an experimental prosthesis to a subject's gait over the course of many days, some research studies have successfully applied an acclimation duration on the order of hours. Herr and Grabowski applied a 2-h span for acclimation in their study featuring a bionic powered prosthesis. This 2-h span encompassed subject adaptation, alignment/fitting, and parameter tuning. For a majority of the walking velocities significant difference regarding metabolic energy cost was discovered for people with transtibial amputation by comparison of the bionic powered prosthesis and passive-elastic prosthesis. Another finding of the study was no significant difference for metabolic energy while contrast the subjects using the bionic powered prosthesis and people without amputation (Herr and Grabowski 2012).

Another study by Mancinelli et al. applied a 1-h acclimation period for their research study. The study pertained to the use of a powered prosthesis, and subjects were permitted to request additional acclimation time. Mancinelli et al. advocated that metabolic cost and biomechanics would reveal a more prominent quantified disparity with the application of a more protracted acclimation duration (Mancinelli et al. 2011).

In consideration of the analysis of the efficacy of previous experimental advanced prosthesis studies, a 2-h minimal threshold is recommended. Greater acclimation periods are recommended to better confirm the efficacy of an advanced prosthesis. The maximal acclimation threshold should be established at the discretion of the research team in consideration of the economies of the endeavor (LeMoyne 2015).

4.16 Alignment of the Prosthesis

The alignment procedure for personalizing a transtibial prosthesis to a person with amputation is critical for the research study and quality of life in terms of personal usage. The role of a certified prosthetist is inherent to experimental research regarding experimental prostheses. A prosthetist is tasked with providing subject specific fitting and alignment (Mancinelli et al. 2011; Herr and Grabowski 2012; LeMoyne 2015).

Sustainable loading patterns, such as about the knee joints, are enabled with an appropriate alignment. Correctly aligning a prosthesis with a subject's unique characteristics can facilitate metabolic efficiency. Of upmost importance the alignment procedure provides a person with amputation with comfortable usage, which is a major quality of life issue (Blumentritt et al. 1999).

By contrast, an incorrectly aligned prosthesis can lead to chronic degeneration about the knee joint. Misalignment can induce the plasticity of adverse muscle activity patterns in an attempt to adapt and stabilize joints. Metabolic cost can be amplified relative to a proper alignment (Blumentritt et al. 1999). Intuitively the event of a misaligned prosthesis can cause a considerably uncomfortable prosthetic experience. Even with the most state of the art powered prosthesis, misalignment can severely obfuscate the quality of the usage experience.

The role of the prosthetist requires a significant level of expertise and acuity. The process for aligning a prosthesis is intrinsically time consuming. The procedure is also subjective in nature. A quantified, objective, and more rapid process with automation would be of considerable interest (Blumentritt et al. 1999).

A technique for aligning a prosthesis with an associated automated feedback process is the Laser Assisted Static Alignment Reference (LASAR) Posture system. The system features a quantified strategy. The LASAR Posture system determines the ground reaction force vertical component. The essential components of the device are the force plate and a motion controlled laser actuated by a stepper motor. The line emanated by the laser projects the center of pressure upon the subject. The laser projection provides visual projection of the center of pressure respective of important anatomical positions about the body, such as joints. The displacement between the laser induced load line is relative to an anatomical feature of prosthetist's preference. The spatial relationship between the laser induced load line and the subject's body enables a useful quantified feedback metric for the prosthetic alignment procedure (Blumentritt 1997).

Conclusion

The assembly of a cohesive test and evaluation strategy is essential to assess the efficacy of a novel powered prosthesis. The biomechanics of gait can be ascertained by kinematic and kinetic variables that can be derived by integrated equipment, such as an optical motion capture system and force plates. Electromyogram and metabolic analyzers can measure muscle activation patterns and metabolic efficiency trends. Recent developments have demonstrated the benefits of wireless and mobile sensor platforms with the application of smartphone and portable media devices to quantify gait patterns. The resulting data can be synthesized into a feature set for machine learning classification, which represents an evolution from acquiring statistical significance. Machine learning classification accuracy represents the eventual capability to derive diagnostic inferences based on quantified gait analysis results. Fundamental aspects of prosthetic testing and evaluation, such as prosthetic alignment procedure and acclimation timeframe, are discussed in order to provide a global perspective.

References

Aldridge JM, Sturdy JT, Wilken JM (2012) Stair ascent kinematics and kinetics with a powered lower leg system following transtibial amputation. Gait Posture 36:291–295

Begg R, Kamruzzaman J (2005) A machine learning approach for automated recognition of movement patterns using basic, kinetic and kinematic gait data. J Biomech 38:401–408

Bland M (2000) An introduction to medical statistics. Oxford University Press, New York

Blumentritt S (1997) A new biomechanical method for determination of static prosthetic alignment. Prosthet Orthot Int 21:107–113

Blumentritt S, Schmalz T, Jarasch R, Schneider M (1999) Effects of sagittal plane prosthetic alignment on standing transtibial amputees knee loads. Prosthet Orthot Int 23:231–238

Brockway JM (1987) Derivation of formulae used to calculate energy expenditure in man. Hum Nutr Clin Nutr 41:463–471

Darter BJ, Wilken JM (2014) Energetic consequences of using a prosthesis with adaptive ankle motion during slope walking in persons with a transtibial amputation. Prosthet Orthot Int 38: 5–11

Dietz V (2002) Proprioception and locomotor disorders. Nat Rev Neurosci 3:781–790

Dobkin BH (2003) The clinical science of neurologic rehabilitation. Oxford University Press, New York

Endo K, Swart E, Herr H (2009) An artificial gastrocnemius for a transtibial prosthesis. Proceedings of 31st annual international conference of the IEEE EMBS, Minneapolis, pp 5034–5037

Fey NP, Klute GK, Neptune RR (2011) The influence of energy storage and return foot stiffness on walking mechanics and muscle activity in below-knee amputees. Clin Biomech 26:1025–1032

Hall M, Frank E, Holmes G, Pfahringer B, Reutemann P, Witten IH (2009) The WEKA data mining software: an update. ACM SIGKDD Explor Newsl 11:10–18

Herr HM, Grabowski AM (2012) Bionic ankle–foot prosthesis normalizes walking gait for persons with leg amputation. Proc Biol Sci 279:457–464

Houdijk H, Pollmann E, Groenewold M, Wiggerts H, Polomski W (2009) The energy cost for the step-to-step transition in amputee walking. Gait Posture 30:35–40

Huston RL (2009) Principles of biomechanics. CRC Press, Boca Raton

ImageJ. http://imagej.nih.gov/ij/index.html

Ishikawa M, Komi PV, Grey MJ, Lepola V, Bruggemann GP (2005) Muscle-tendon interaction and elastic energy usage in human walking. J Appl Physiol 99:603–608

Kinovea. http://www.kinovea.org

LeMoyne R (2015) Advances regarding powered prosthesis for transtibial amputation. J Mech Med Biol 15:1–34

LeMoyne R, Mastroianni T (2012) iWalk, a gait analysis device incorporating an iPod wireless accelerometer application. 42nd Annual Society for Neuroscience, New Orleans

LeMoyne R, Mastroianni T (2015) Use of smartphones and portable media devices for quantifying human movement characteristics of gait, tendon reflex response, and Parkinson's disease hand tremor, chap 23. In: Rasooly A, Herold KE (eds) Mobile health technologies: methods and protocols. Springer, New York

LeMoyne R, Coroian C, Mastroianni T, Grundfest W (2008a) Virtual proprioception. J Mech Med Biol 8:317–338

LeMoyne R, Coroian C, Mastroianni T, Grundfest W (2008b) Accelerometers for quantification of gait and movement disorders: a perspective review. J Mech Med Biol 8:137–152

LeMoyne R, Coroian C, Mastroianni T, Wu W, Grundfest W, Kaiser W (2008c) Virtual proprioception with real-time step detection and processing. Proceedings of 30th annual international conference of the IEEE EMBS, Vancouver, pp 4238–4241

LeMoyne R, Coroian C, Mastroianni T, Opalinski P, Cozza M, Grundfest W (2009a) The merits of artificial proprioception, with applications in biofeedback gait rehabilitation concepts and movement disorder characterization, chap 10. In: Barros de Mello CA (ed) Biomedical engineering. Intech, Vienna

LeMoyne R, Coroian C, Mastroianni T, Grundfest W (2009b) Wireless accelerometer assessment of gait for quantified disparity of hemiparetic locomotion. J Mech Med Biol 9:329–343

LeMoyne R, Mastroianni T, Cozza M, Coroian C, Grundfest W (2010a) Implementation of an iPhone as a wireless accelerometer for quantifying gait characteristics. Proceedings of 32nd annual international conference of the IEEE EMBS, Buenos Aires, pp 3847–3851

LeMoyne R, Mastroianni T, Cozza M, Coroian C (2010b) iPhone wireless accelerometer application for acquiring quantified gait attributes. Proceedings of ASME 2010 5th frontiers in biomedical devices conference, Newport Beach, pp 19–20

LeMoyne R, Mastroianni T, Cozza M, Coroian C (2010c) Quantification of gait characteristics through a functional iPhone wireless accelerometer application mounted to the spine. Proceedings of ASME 2010 5th frontiers in biomedical devices conference, Newport Beach, pp 87–88

LeMoyne R, Mastroianni T, Grundfest W (2011) Wireless accelerometer iPod application for quantifying gait characteristics. Proceedings of 33rd annual international conference of the IEEE EMBS, Boston, pp 7904–7907

LeMoyne R, Mastroianni T, Grundfest W (2013) Wireless accelerometer system for quantifying disparity of hemiplegic gait using the frequency domain. J Mech Med Biol 13:1–19

LeMoyne R, Mastroianni T, Montoya K (2014a) Implementation of a smartphone for evaluating gait characteristics of a trans-tibial prosthesis. Proceedings of 36th annual international conference of the IEEE EMBS, Chicago, pp 3674–3677

LeMoyne R, Kerr W, Mastroianni T, Hessel A (2014b) Implementation of machine learning for classifying hemiplegic gait disparity through use of a force plate. Proceedings of 13th international conference on machine learning and applications (ICMLA), Detroit, pp 379–382

LeMoyne R, Mastroianni T, Hessel A, Nishikawa K (2015a) Implementation of machine learning for classifying prosthesis type through conventional gait analysis. Proceedings of 37th annual international conference of the IEEE EMBS, Milan, pp 202–205

LeMoyne R, Mastroianni T, Tomycz N, Whiting D, McCandless C, Peduto D, Cozza M (2015b) I-Phone wireless accelerometer quantification of extremity tremor in essential tremor patient undergoing activated and inactivated deep brain stimulation. Proceedings of international neuromodulation society's 12th world congress, Montréal

LeMoyne R, Tomycz N, Mastroianni T, McCandless C, Cozza M, Peduto D (2015c) Implementation of a smartphone wireless accelerometer platform for establishing deep brain stimulation treatment efficacy of essential tremor with machine learning. Proceedings of 37th annual international conference of the IEEE EMBS, Milan, pp 6772–6775

Levinger P, Lai DT, Webster K, Begg RK, Feller J (2007) Support vector machines for detecting recovery from knee replacement surgery using quantitative gait measures. Proceedings of 29th annual international conference of the IEEE EMBS, Lyon, pp 4875–4878

Levinger P, Lai DT, Begg RK, Webster KE, Feller JA (2009) The application of support vector machines for detecting recovery from knee replacement surgery using spatio-temporal gait parameters. Gait Posture 29:91–96

Mancinelli C, Patritti BL, Tropea P, Greenwald RM, Casler R, Herr H, Bonato P (2011) Comparing a passive-elastic and a powered prosthesis in transtibial amputees. Proceedings of 33rd annual international conference of the IEEE EMBS, Boston, pp 8255–8258

Morgenroth DC, Segal AD, Zelik KE, Czerniecki JM, Klute GK, Adamczyk PG, Orendurff MS, Hahn ME, Collins SH, Kuo AD (2011) The effect of prosthetic foot push-off on mechanical loading associated with knee osteoarthritis in lower extremity amputees. Gait Posture 34: 502–507

Okada H, Ae M, Robertson DG (2007) The effect of ground reaction force components on ankle joint torque during walking. J Biomech 40:S511

Perry J (1992) Gait analysis: normal and pathological function. Slack, Thorofare

Ryall NH, Eyres SB, Neumann VC, Bhakta BB, Tennant A (2003) The SIGAM mobility grades: a new population-specific measure for lower limb amputees. Disabil Rehabil 25:833–844

Saremi K, Marehbian J, Yan X, Regnaux JP, Elashoff R, Bussel B, Dobkin BH (2006) Reliability and validity of bilateral thigh and foot accelerometry measures of walking in healthy and hemiparetic subjects. Neurorehabil Neural Repair 20:297–305

Savelberg HH, de Lange AL (1999) Assessment of the horizontal, fore-aft component of the ground reaction force from insole pressure patterns by using artificial neural networks. Clin Biomech 14:585–592

Tracker. http://www.cabrillo.edu/~dbrown/tracker/

Weka. http://www.cs.waikato.ac.nz/~ml/weka/

Wilson AB Jr (1963) Prosthetics and orthotics research in the United States. Orthop Prosthet Appli J 17:152–160

Winter DA (1990) Biomechanics and motor control of human movement. Wiley-Interscience, New York

Witten IH, Frank E, Hall MA (2011) Data mining: practical machine learning tools and techniques. Morgan Kaufmann, Burlington

Chapter 5
Passive Transtibial Prosthesis and Associated Prosthetic Components

Abstract The foundation to the evolution pathways of the transtibial prosthesis is the passive prosthesis. The origins of the passive prosthesis date on the scale of centuries prior to current. Although a passive prosthesis is not in general capable of providing elastic or mechanized energy to the terminal aspects of stance phase of gait, there are still reasons for why the passive prosthesis is still currently implemented. Passive prostheses serve as robust alternatives in challenging environmental settings, and they constitute a feasible contingency for developing countries. Regardless of the specific class of transtibial prosthesis, there exist associated prosthetic components, such as a socket, liner, and pylon. The socket represents the interface between the prosthesis and the residual limb. Between the socket and residual limb exists a liner that generally consists of an energy absorbing medium. The socket and liner are critical for properly fitting the prosthesis to the unique and specific requirements of a person with an amputation. Between the socket and ankle-foot assembly resides the pylon. The pylon generally enables structural support through conventional metallic materials. Recently, geographically localized materials, such as bamboo, have been incorporated as pylons. The foundations of the passive prosthesis, such as the Solid Ankle Cushioned Heel (SACH), provide a significant perspective for the design evolution of the prosthetic technology. A comprehension of the utility of the socket, liner, and pylon enable a synergistic prosthetic design.

Keywords Passive prosthesis • Socket • Liner • Pylon • Prosthetic interface

5.1 Introduction

The transtibial prosthesis has undergone considerable evolution. Original functional prostheses for attempting to enable gait served the role of providing structural support (Fey et al. 2011; LeMoyne 2015). Such designs are exemplified by the endeavor of Paré. This version of the transtibial prosthesis is generally the most basic from an historical perspective (LeMoyne 2015).

The most fundamental prosthesis for persons with transtibial amputation is the Solid Ankle Cushioned Heel (SACH) (May and Lockard 2011; LeMoyne 2015). This type of prosthesis was developed in response to focused research and

R. LeMoyne, *Advances for Prosthetic Technology*,
DOI 10.1007/978-4-431-55816-3_5

development at the institutional level from the United States of America (Wilson 1963). The SACH is designed from rigid material, such as a lightweight metal, and the base of the prosthesis is cushioned with a material, such as rubber. The advantage of the SACH is established in consideration of the simplicity of its design. The inexpensive and low maintenance nature of the SACH makes it highly attractive for developing nations with limited economies for their healthcare system (Wilson 1963; Meanley 1995; Day 1996; Jensen and Heim 1999; LeMoyne 2015).

The inherent nature of the SACH in light of its selected material is that it is effectively non-responsive throughout the gait cycle. The SACH provides minimal energy return during the stance phase of the gait cycle. The SACH is also not capable of modulating ankle angular orientation during swing phase (Wilson 1963; May and Lockard 2011; LeMoyne 2015).

In consideration of the number of average steps a person takes throughout only a day and furthermore a year, an assortment of lower limb morbidities can logically develop (Burke et al. 1978; Nolan et al. 2003; Mündermann et al. 2005; Morgenroth et al. 2011, 2012; LeMoyne 2015). During the 1980s Winters discovered that plantar flexion musculature during the stance phase provides roughly 80 % of the mechanical power to the entire gait cycle (Winter 1983; Winter and Sienko 1988; Sanderson and Martin 1997; Dobkin 2003; LeMoyne 2015). As a transtibial amputation removes this feature of the gait cycle, gait asymmetries, which could lead to long-term issues, such as osteoarthritis about lower limb joints (Burke et al. 1978; Nolan et al. 2003; Mündermann et al. 2005; Morgenroth et al. 2011, 2012; LeMoyne 2015). Another disadvantage of the SACH is the lack of controlling ankle orientation during swing phase, which can lead to potential for toe-drag and possible falling.

Two other classes of transtibial prosthesis have been recently developed to ameliorate the SACH's inability to contribute energy during the stance phase of gait. Since the 1980s Energy Storage and Return (ESAR) prostheses have been developed (Burgess et al. 1985). The concept of the ESAR involves modifying the material selection for the prosthesis, such that energy can be stored upon stance initiation and released during the terminal phase (Burgess et al. 1985; Fey et al. 2011). The energy storing and releasing material can reside in the foot ankle assembly or also integral with the pylon that extends from the prosthetic socket interface to the foot ankle assembly (Burgess et al. 1985; Michael 1987). More recent evolutions of the ESAR have incorporated mechatronics to control the timing of the stored energy release (LeMoyne 2015). Due to the conservation of energy the ESAR can only release a limited amount of stored potential energy, and they are generally more complex and expensive relative to the SACH (Serway 1990; LeMoyne 2015).

The most advanced prosthesis is the powered prosthesis that imparts mechanical energy about the stance phase through a robotically actuated system. The class is the most technologically advanced. However it is also the most expensive and complex prosthetic scheme (LeMoyne 2015; BiOM). As manufacturing of these systems increases, their expense will likely decrease.

The ESAR and most advanced powered prostheses are reserved for future chapters, such as Chap. 6: 'Energy Storage and Return (ESAR) prosthesis', Chap. 8: 'Transtibial powered prostheses: single and dual actuator configurations', and Chap. 9: 'The MIT inspired powered prosthesis leading to the commercialized BiOM powered prosthesis, a precedence in transtibial prosthetic technology'. This chapter emphasizes the role of the SACH and supporting components, such as the socket, liner, and suspension. The significance of the supporting components is ubiquitous and universal for all classes of transtibial prosthesis. These components serve a significant role for the overall quality of the prosthetic system. From a failure mode effect analysis perspective from the system level, any issues with the functional efficacy of these components can severely impact the entire prosthetic application. Therefore, primary component level aspects globally applied for a prosthetic system are featured in this chapter.

The global prosthetic system for a transtibial amputee consists of multiple components that each serves an integral function. A prosthetic system must comfortably interface with the subject's residual limb of the leg. The interface is achieved from a custom socket, which incorporates a liner to provide cushioning and support between the residual leg and socket. As the residual limb of the leg is not intended for load bearing, the features of the socket and liner substantially impact a transtibial subject's quality of life. The interface between the prosthetic system and residual limb are supported by a suspension component that sustains a connectivity between the prosthesis and residual limb. The integrity of the suspension can literally represent the difference between a prosthesis remaining attached during gait and sliding off the subject's residual limb. Following the socket is the pylon that can represent the tibia-fibula skeletal structure. The pylon must be designed with material capable of sustaining the inherent repetitive stress of walking. Such pylons connect with ankle-heel emulating devices, such as the SACH (May and Lockard 2011; LeMoyne 2015). These components for the basic prosthesis warrant further description.

5.2 Socket

The socket constitutes the interface medium between the prosthesis and subject's residual limb. Each socket is uniquely adapted to the subject, and prosthetist's acuity and experience considerably influence the capacity to customize the socket to the subject's requirements. The development of a socket is influenced by factors, such as amputation level and spatial characteristics of the residual limb (May and Lockard 2011).

The fundamental of the socket design is to enable body weight support. The socket should also enable a reliable interface with the prosthesis, while not compromising the perceived comfort for a subject's desired activity level. As the global objective of a prosthetic is to enable functional restoration of gait, a firm fit to the residual limb mitigates the movement of the socket relative to the residual limb skin. The patellar tendon bearing socket is commonly used for subjects with transtibial amputation (May and Lockard 2011).

As subject unique socket can be enabled by modern scanning techniques and computational strategies. These technologies enable resources to be remotely situated as stored data may be easily conveyed through Internet connectivity. A laser digital scanner records the topology of a subject's residual limb. With the spatial features of the residual limb defined in a 3-dimensional context, the images can be conveyed to manufacturing for fabrication of the socket (May and Lockard 2011).

This new strategy demonstrates the evolution of biomedical technology. Past techniques incorporate the creation of a cast about the residual limb. With the cast, a positive mold can be developed for subsequent fabrication of the socket. Multiple advantages are demonstrated by the modern technique incorporating laser digital scanning. A reduction in disposable materials is apparent, as laser scanning does not require a cast or positive mold. The non-contact nature of the modern technique may also ameliorate any discomfort and risk of infection for a person adapting to a recent amputation (May and Lockard 2011).

An amputated residual limb is not intended for the repetitive load bearing of gait and other activities. There can exist areas of the residual limb that are highly sensitive to pressure loading, such as sharp protrusions of bone from the tibia and fibula and neural projections, such as from the peroneal nerve that are proximal to the skin (Silver-Thorn et al. 1996; May and Lockard 2011; LeMoyne 2015).

By contrast, pressure tolerant tissues are demonstrated by tendons and flat structures of bone. Patellar tendon bearing sockets predominantly incorporate the concept of total surface bearing. The objective of this concept is to distribute pressure throughout the pressure tolerant aspects of the residual limb (May and Lockard 2011).

5.3 Liner

Between the socket and residual limb exists a sock, which also incorporates a liner. The liner consists of energy-absorbing and cushioning gel material. Although the liner enables cushioning, shear forces inherent with the interface between residual limb and socket are not ameliorated (May and Lockard 2011).

Since the mid-1980s the application of the silicon liner has become more prevalent for transtibial prosthesis applications. From a material perspective silicon is characterized as a flexible and adhesive medium. This enables the silicon liner to comply with the contour of the residual limb contour. These capabilities enable the residual limb stump to conform with the total surface bearing perspective that occurs while loading the prosthesis. Symmetric loading occurs during stance phase of gait and standing, such that pressure is effectively evenly distributed (Kristinsson 1993; Baars and Geertzen 2005). By enabling a superior fit about the socket a subject can experience advances in proprioception, which can enhance overall prosthetic performance (Baars and Geertzen 2005).

In general Baars and Geertzen advocate the use of silicon liners for transtibial prosthesis. Findings support the claim that liners facilitate the suspension mechanism of the prosthesis. Improving gait performance facilitates a subject's activity patterns while ameliorating dependence on assistive devices (Baars and Geertzen 2005).

5.4 Suspension

The quality of the suspension component diminishes shear forces intrinsic with the limb-socket interface. This movement occurrence is referred to as pistoning. Especially for active subjects such adverse movement can cause skin abrasions leading to discomfort (Michael 2004; May and Lockard 2011; Gholizadeh et al. 2012). Such morbidities can naturally impair a subject's functional capacity.

Suspension components that incorporate suction have been demonstrated as an efficacious means for eliminating pistoning between the limb and socket. This scheme is achieved by developing a vacuum. The vacuum is sustained by a one-way valve that expels air from between the socket and residual limb (Klute et al. 2011; May and Lockard 2011; Gholizadeh et al. 2014a).

There are major two configurations: the valve and sleeve and valve integrated with liner. The valve and liner configuration amalgamates the expulsion valve with the sealed liner. The valve and sleeve incorporates an expulsion valve with a suction sleeve that mounts above the liner above the liner. The devices are expensive and are often replaced. They also inherently implicate issues regarding thermal retention and perspiration. Clear benefits involve elimination of pistoning and reliable suspension. These features also enable augmented limb control and enhanced proprioception (May and Lockard 2011; Gholizadeh et al. 2014b).

5.5 Pylon

For the most fundamental prosthesis, the pylon is the structure between the socket and the ankle-foot ankle assembly of the prosthetic system. The pylon enables structural and geometric (length) characteristics for the prosthetic system. A pylon functions as a load bearing structure similar in role to the tibula-fibula bones of the skeleton. It extends from the socket to the foot ankle assembly. An array of materials can satisfy the requirements for the pylon component (Seymour 2002).

The pylon primarily consists of metals. The selected material for a transtibial prosthesis pylon is specific to the preferences and characteristics of the subject. Three major types of metallic pylons are:

- stainless steel
- titanium
- aluminum (Scherer et al. 1999; Seymour 2002; Shasmin et al. 2008a)

Titanium offers a highly lightweight alternative (Seymour 2002). Stainless steel and aluminum are intuitively less expensive. Recently Shasmin et al. conducted a study that compared the biomechanical features of stainless steel pylons to pylons consisting of bamboo. The findings revealed no significant differences respective of gait kinematic properties, such as cadence and stride velocity, between the two materials (Shasmin et al. 2008a).

Bamboo offers a novel alternative to traditional metallic pylons. This new perspective for below knee prosthetic design may be highly useful for developing countries residing in locations where bamboo constitutes a highly abundant natural resources, such as South America and Asia. Preliminary testing and evaluation has demonstrated that bamboo offers superior specific strength relative to conventional pylon materials, such as aluminum. As bamboo constitutes a recently addressed alternative for the pylon assembly of a lower leg prosthesis, more testing and evaluation is imperative. For example, dynamic characteristics and material life-time should be better defined (Shasmin et al. 2008b).

5.6 Solid Ankle Cushioned Heel (SACH)

The most basic prosthesis for transtibial amputation involves the solid ankle cushioned heel, which is commonly abbreviated as SACH. The SACH is an inherently passive prosthetic. The principal benefit that the SACH enables is structural support that is an imperative requirement about the stance phase of gait (Fey et al. 2011; LeMoyne 2015).

Since the SACH is comprised of passive components, it intuitively lacks the capacity to adapt to gait perturbations that are an essential aspect of robust walking. Minimal energy is conserved during the stance phase. As a consequence, this lack of energy imparted during stance leads to an amplified metabolic cost that constitutes a major quality of life impairment during prolonged walking (Au et al. 2007a, b; Au 2007; Fey et al. 2011; LeMoyne 2015).

Another consequence of transtibial passive prosthetic is the development of gait asymmetries. These asymmetries in a repetitive and prolonged context can degenerate to chronic morbidities, causing further duress to quality of life (Au et al. 2007a, b; Au 2007; Fey et al. 2011; LeMoyne 2015). Logically the obvious benefits of prosthetic technologies that can release energy and even generate work for the gait cycle can be currently deduced. In order for the modern engineer to be able to evolve the current state of the art of prosthetic technology, a perspective on the evolution that led to the SACH and its continuance for the course of multiple decades should be considered.

A visual inspection of the first substantive kind of transtibial prosthesis developed by Paré reveals the most obvious restoration of structural and load bearing function for people with lower limb amputation (Thurston 2007; Hernigou 2013; LeMoyne 2015). Centuries later Hanger employed materials in his designs for lower limb prostheses that incorporated rubber bumpers for improving emulation of the ankle-foot complex during stance phase of gait (May and Lockard 2011). Later after the Second World War and entire ensemble of top American engineers and scientists contributed to the development of the SACH (Wilson 1963). Until a better comprehension of the significant contribution of the ankle-foot complex during stance phase, the prevalent usage of the SACH persisted (May and Lockard 2011; LeMoyne 2015).

Major scientific findings for the features of human gait have been elucidated over the course of the past few decades, which have promoted further advances of lower limb prostheses (LeMoyne 2015). For example, the substantial contribution of powered plantar flexion to the gait cycle imparted during stance was discovered by the research of Winter (Winter 1983; Winter and Sienko 1988; Sanderson and Martin 1997; Dobkin 2003; LeMoyne 2015). Therefore, the need for imparting energy to the stance phase of gait, whether by actuator or material elasticity, has been a topic of considerable interest (Au et al. 2007a; Au 2007; Zelik 2012; Grimmer and Seyfarth 2014; LeMoyne 2015). The discoveries encompassing the neurology of gait has led to the findings of the significance of neurological structures, such as the central pattern generator, that modulates gait and greatly improves responsiveness (Kandel et al. 2000; Dietz 2002; LeMoyne et al. 2008; Watson et al. 2010). Current emulations of computerized prosthetic platforms have emulated reflexes, a critical aspect of the lower limb neurology (Eilenberg et al. 2010; Markowitz et al. 2011; LeMoyne 2015).

Although developed countries with considerable economic resources that equip their healthcare system can provide expensive lower limb prostheses for their people. For people with lower limb amputations in developing countries the requirements are logically influenced by the apparent limitations of economic resources. With more challenged healthcare economies developing countries are generally predisposed toward more simplified prosthetic alternatives, such as the SACH approach.

With respect to developing countries, establishing the proper type of prosthetic technology is major challenge. The prosthesis design requirements are unique to the environmental constraints. A simple alternative enables an appropriate utility. Developing countries therefore strongly favor the SACH (Meanley 1995; Day 1996; Jensen and Heim 1999). The SACH model is also favored as local materials can manufacture it (Meanley 1995). For example, Vietnam has produced SACH prostheses through internal manufacturing resources (Jensen and Heim 1999). This pragmatism underscores the perspective that a state of the art powered prosthesis serves minimal utility for people with amputation residing rural to a primary city in an environment, such as a tropical rainforest setting.

Although SACH prostheses have become more prevalent in developing countries and less frequently prescribed in developed countries, a notable trend in technological evolution should be observed. The SACH was a research and development inspiration from the National Academy of Sciences instilled by the Committee on Prosthetics Research and Development of the United States of America, which is a highly developed nation (Wilson 1963). However, on the order of a half century later, this design highly preferred in developing countries (Meanley 1995; Day 1996; Jensen and Heim 1999). The observation of these trends is that current research and development technologies, such as the powered prosthesis, should also eventually permeate developing countries.

Conclusion

The evolutionary trend of the transtibial prosthesis originates from load-bearing and primarily structural tasked designs, such as the Solid Ankle Cushioned Heel (SACH) prosthesis. With the role of the plantar flexors of the lower limb well established during the later 1980s, the objective shifted toward the developing prostheses capable of imparting energy about the stance phase of gait, either through energy absorbing elasticity with subsequent release or powered actuation.

All of these prosthetic application strategies share the commonality of the need to interface the residual limb to the prescribed prosthesis. A custom made socket is uniquely designed for the subject, individualizing function and comfort. A liner enables further comfort about the interface with improvements in energy absorption quality. The suspension serves the critical role of securing the prosthesis, especially during gait, while minimizing pistoning, which may severely impair a subject's quality of life.

Before comprehensively addressing the powered prosthesis strategy, the next aspect of the evolutionary continuum for prosthetic technology shall be encompassed in the following Chap. 6: 'Energy Storage and Return (ESAR) prosthesis'. The Energy Storage and Return (ESAR) prosthesis incorporates a select material that is capable of storing potential energy during stance phase onset and releasing the energy on the more terminal aspects of stance. One type of prosthesis that first satisfied these design criteria is the Seattle Foot.

References

Au SK (2007) Powered ankle-foot prosthesis for the improvement of amputee walking economy. Ph.D. dissertation, MIT, Department of Mechanical Engineering, Cambridge

Au SK, Herr H, Weber J, Martinez-Villalpando EC (2007a) Powered ankle-foot prosthesis for the improvement of amputee ambulation. Proceedings of 29th annual international conference of the IEEE EMBS, Lyon, pp 3020–3026

Au SK, Weber J, Herr H (2007b) Biomechanical design of a powered ankle-foot prosthesis. Proceedings of IEEE 10th international conference on rehabilitation robotics, Noordwijk, pp 298–303

Baars EC, Geertzen JH (2005) Literature review of the possible advantages of silicon liner socket use in trans-tibial prostheses. Prosthet Orthot Int 29:27–37

BiOM. www.biom.com; www.bionxmed.com

Burgess EM, Poggi DL, Hittenberger DA, Zettl JH, Moeller DE, Carpenter KL, Forsgren SM (1985) Development and preliminary evaluation of the VA Seattle foot. J Rehabil Res Dev 22:75–84
Burke MJ, Roman V, Wright V (1978) Bone and joint changes in lower limb amputees. Ann Rheum Dis 37:252–254
Day HJ (1996) A review of the consensus conference on appropriate prosthetic technology in developing countries. Prosthet Orthot Int 20:15–23
Dietz V (2002) Proprioception and locomotor disorders. Nat Rev Neurosci 3:781–790
Dobkin BH (2003) The clinical science of neurologic rehabilitation. Oxford University Press, New York
Eilenberg MF, Geyer H, Herr H (2010) Control of a powered ankle–foot prosthesis based on a neuromuscular model. IEEE Trans Neural Syst Rehabil Eng 18:164–173
Fey NP, Klute GK, Neptune RR (2011) The influence of energy storage and return foot stiffness on walking mechanics and muscle activity in below-knee amputees. Clin Biomech 26:1025–1032
Gholizadeh H, Abu Osman NA, Eshraghi A, Ali S, Sævarsson SK, Wan Abas WA, Pirouzi GH (2012) Transtibial prosthetic suspension: less pistoning versus easy donning and doffing. J Rehabil Res Dev 49:1321–1330
Gholizadeh H, Abu Osman NA, Eshraghi A, Ali S, Razak NA (2014a) Transtibial prosthesis suspension systems: systematic review of literature. Clin Biomech 29:87–97
Gholizadeh H, Abu Osman NA, Eshraghi A, Ali S, Arifin N, Abas WA (2014b) Evaluation of new suspension system for limb prosthetics. Biomed Eng Online 13:1–13
Grimmer M, Seyfarth A (2014) Mimicking human-like leg function in prosthetic limbs, chap 5. In: Artemiadis P (ed) Neuro-robotics: from brain machine interfaces to rehabilitation robotics. Springer, Dordrecht
Hernigou P (2013) Ambroise Paré IV: the early history of artificial limbs (from robotic to prostheses). Int Orthop 37:1195–1197
Jensen JS, Heim S (1999) Preliminary experiences with modified SACH feet manufactured and used in a tropical developing world setting. Prosthet Orthot Int 23:245–248
Kandel ER, Schwartz JH, Jessell TM (2000) Principles of neural science. McGraw-Hill, New York
Klute GK, Berge JS, Biggs W, Pongnumkul S, Popovic Z, Curless B (2011) Vacuum-assisted socket suspension compared with pin suspension for lower extremity amputees: effect on fit, activity, and limb volume. Arch Phys Med Rehabil 92:1570–1575
Kristinsson Ö (1993) The ICEROSS concept: a discussion of a philosophy. Prosthet Orthot Int 17:49–55
LeMoyne R (2015) Advances regarding powered prosthesis for transtibial amputation. J Mech Med Biol 15:1–34
LeMoyne R, Coroian C, Mastroianni T, Grundfest W (2008) Virtual proprioception. J Mech Med Biol 8:317–338
Markowitz J, Krishnaswamy P, Eilenberg MF, Endo K, Barnhart C, Herr H (2011) Speed adaptation in a powered transtibial prosthesis controlled with a neuromuscular model. Philos Trans R Soc Lond B Biol Sci 366:1621–1631
May BJ, Lockard MA (2011) Prosthetics & orthotics in clinical practice: a case study approach. FA Davis, Philadelphia
Meanley S (1995) Different approaches and cultural considerations in third world prosthetics. Prosthet Orthot Int 19:176–180
Michael J (1987) Energy storing feet: a clinical comparison. Clin Prosthet Orthot 11:154–168
Michael JW (2004) Prosthetic suspensions and components. In: Smith DG, Michael JW, Bowker JH (eds) Atlas of amputations and limb deficiencies: surgical, prosthetic, and rehabilitation principles. American Academy of Orthopaedic Surgeons, Rosemont, pp 409–425
Morgenroth DC, Segal AD, Zelik KE, Czerniecki JM, Klute GK, Adamczyk PG, Orendurff MS, Hahn ME, Collins SH, Kuo AD (2011) The effect of prosthetic foot push-off on mechanical loading associated with knee osteoarthritis in lower extremity amputees. Gait Posture 34:502–507

Morgenroth DC, Gellhorn AC, Suri P (2012) Osteoarthritis in the disabled population: a mechanical perspective. PM R 4:S20–S27
Mündermann A, Dyrby CO, Andriacchi TP (2005) Secondary gait changes in patients with medial compartment knee osteoarthritis: increased load at the ankle, knee, and hip during walking. Arthritis Rheum 52:2835–2844
Nolan L, Wit A, Dudziñski K, Lees A, Lake M, Wychowañski M (2003) Adjustments in gait symmetry with walking speed in trans-femoral and trans-tibial amputees. Gait Posture 17:142–151
Sanderson DJ, Martin PE (1997) Lower extremity kinematic and kinetic adaptations in unilateral - below-knee amputees during walking. Gait Posture 6:126–136
Scherer RF, Dowling JJ, Frost G, Robinson M, McLean K (1999) Mechanical and metabolic work of persons with lower-extremity amputations walking with titanium and stainless steel prostheses: a preliminary study. J Prosthet Orthot 11:38–42
Serway RA (1990) Physics for scientists and engineers. Saunders College, Philadelphia
Seymour R (2002) Prosthetics and orthotics: lower limb and spinal. Lippincott Williams & Wilkins, Philadelphia
Shasmin HN, Abu Osman NA, Latif LA (2008a) Comparison between biomechanical characteristics of stainless steel and bamboo pylons: a preliminary study. Proceedings of 4th Kuala Lumpur international conference on biomedical engineering, Kuala Lumpur, pp 851–853
Shasmin HN, Abu Osman NA, Latif LA (2008b) Economical tube adapter material in below knee prosthesis. Proceedings of 4th Kuala Lumpur international conference on biomedical engineering, Kuala Lumpur, pp 407–409
Silver-Thorn MB, Steege JW, Childress DS (1996) A review of prosthetic interface stress investigations. J Rehabil Res Dev 33:253–266
Thurston AJ (2007) Paré and prosthetics: the early history of artificial limbs. ANZ J Surg 77:1114–1119
Watson C, Kirkcaldie M, Paxinos G (2010) The brain: an introduction to functional neuroanatomy. Academic Press, New York
Wilson AB Jr (1963) Prosthetics and orthotics research in the United States. Orthop Prosthet Appli J 17:152–160
Winter DA (1983) Energy generation and absorption at the ankle and knee during fast, natural, and slow cadences. Clin Orthop Relat Res 175:147–154
Winter DA, Sienko SE (1988) Biomechanics of below-knee amputee gait. J Biomech 21:361–367
Zelik KE (2012) Passive energy-saving mechanisms in human locomotion. Ph.D. dissertation, University of Michigan, Department of Mechanical Engineering, Ann Arbor

Chapter 6
Energy Storage and Return (ESAR) Prosthesis

Abstract The engineering evolutionary process of the prosthesis for people with transtibial amputation is synergistically linked with relevant scientific discovery regarding the gait cycle. During the 1980s a major breakthrough was made in terms of the role of the ankle-foot complex during the gait cycle. During the terminal aspect of stance phase powered plantar flexion imparts a substantial level of mechanical energy to the gait cycle. In tandem with the decade of this discovery the concept of the Energy Storage and Return (ESAR) prosthesis progressively evolved. Preliminary energy storage and return prostheses incorporated an elastically deflectable keel in the prosthetic foot aspect. This design would store a portion of energy during the impact of stance initiation with a subsequent release during the terminal aspect of stance. Later versions of energy storage and return prostheses would incorporate the effective length from the foot assembly to the socket as energy storing and releasing medium. As the standard energy storage and return prosthesis lacks the capacity to temporally control the release of elastically stored potential energy, the incorporation of mechatronic subsystems facilitated the controlled release of stored energy. The Controlled Energy Storage and Return (CESR) incorporate a microelectronics package and clutch mechanism for controlling the timed release of stored mechanical energy. Prostheses that apply energy storage and return have been the subject of considerable testing and evaluation, which have demonstrated improvements both qualitative for the user and quantitative in terms of gait analysis techniques.

Keywords Energy storage and return prosthesis • Elastic deflection • Conservation of energy • Controlled energy storage and return prosthesis • Mechatronic

6.1 Introduction

During the 1980s a paradigm shift occurred regarding the prosthesis for people with transtibial amputation. The role of the ankle-foot complex became more clearly realized. As the Solid Ankle Cushioned Heel (SACH) prosthesis developed decades before facilitated a semblance of braking with a cushioned heel, the role of powered plantar flexion, which contributes mechanical energy to the gait cycle, became distinctly understood. With the synthesis of these observations, a prosthesis that can

R. LeMoyne, *Advances for Prosthetic Technology*,
DOI 10.1007/978-4-431-55816-3_6

store energy during initiation of stance phase and return a portion of the stored energy back to the gait cycle at the more terminal aspect of stance would constitute a major improvement in prosthetic technology. This type of prosthesis is referred to as an Energy Storage and Return (ESAR) prosthesis (LeMoyne 2015).

The overriding physics that support the energy storage and return prosthesis is the conservation of elastic energy. The initiation of stance cycle imparts a load on the ESAR prosthesis. Rather that providing maximal rigidity such as the solid ankle cushioned heel prosthesis, the energy storage and return prosthesis undergoes a degree of prescribed deflection. A portion of the kinetic energy from the initiation of impact during stance initiation is stored as potential energy, which is released about the terminal aspect of the stance phase (Zelik et al. 2011; Zelik 2012; LeMoyne 2015).

Although the ESAR constitutes an advance relative to the SACH, the ESAR configuration is still limited in terms of performance. Observation of the first law of thermodynamics reveals that only a fractional portion of the kinetic energy stored on stance initiation and stored potential energy can be again released at the final phase of stance. As the ESAR concept entails solely energy storage and release, the degree of energy provided to the gait cycle is constrained by these limitations. Additional kinetic energy cannot be imparted to the gait cycle (Serway 1990; Zelik et al. 2011; Zelik 2012; LeMoyne 2015).

6.2 Seattle Foot

During the mid-1980s an energy storage and return prosthesis called the Seattle Foot was developed. This prosthesis was the result of research and development funding from the United States of America Veterans Administration. The deflecting mechanism that stores energy for pending release is a keel that is encased about a molded rendition of a representative anatomical foot. During the progressive loading of stance phase the keel deflects while storing potential energy. With the forward progress of stance, the energy is progressively released as elastic kinetic energy as weight bearing of the stance phase attenuates (Burgess et al. 1985).

The deflection of the keel is predetermined as a function of subject weight and material properties. Preliminary versions that led to the Seattle Foot incorporated fiberglass integrated with light metal. The design perspective emphasized minimizing parts, so that cost could be reduced and maintenance simplified. Also a monolithic keel was foreseen to provide a more uniform response. Based on these preferences the material Delrin was selected to represent the monolithic keel (Burgess et al. 1985).

Initial clinical evaluation emphasized categorical classification interpreted by the subjects, especially relative to their previous prosthetic foot. The subjects noted relatively considerable ease regarding walking and running. Subjects believed they could engage in greater athletic activity, and overall they considered the Seattle Foot to constitute an improvement compared to their previous prosthesis by a wide margin (Burgess et al. 1985). Underscoring the impact of the Seattle Foot, its evolutions are still currently applied (Seattle Foot).

Further testing and evaluation was conducted by Reswick. This version of the Seattle Foot utilized the similar principle of the deflecting keel (leafspring) during stance loading providing the subject with some restorative push during terminal stance. The keel consisted of a plastic, which was encapsulated in a foam signifying a cosmetic foot. Subjects noted enhancement of gait velocity and more responsive agility (Reswick 1986).

Preliminary life cycle testing was conducted through a loading device to simulate stance phase of walking. Testing and evaluation incorporated a sock and shoe of United States of America military standard. Pressure was adjusted to represent a 175 pound subject. A total of 500,000 loading cycles were applied, and within every 25,000 cycles the Seattle Foot was dismounted, uncovered, and examined for failures. The visual inspection of all samples were determined similar both prior and subsequent to the 500,000 loading cycles. This life cycle test was considered more severe compared to typical use, because the continual loading patterns could even lead to energy storage increase and associated thermal effects (Reswick 1986).

The findings of Reswick underscore the significance of the context of a prosthetic application. A more mechanically complex prosthetic system may not be able to endure 500,000 loading cycles as robustly as the Seattle Foot. User environmental scenarios logically exist that would infer this type of energy storage and return prosthesis is preferable. Also, economic considerations may advocate a more robust and simple prosthesis in light of the usage context.

6.3 Flex-Foot

Proximal to the time frame that the Seattle Foot was developed, another team of researchers created the Flex-Foot. This design perspective significantly differs from the Seattle Foot in multiple approaches. This prosthesis is constructed of graphite composite, which is lightweight with improved mass distribution properties. Flex-Foots are uniquely crafted to the subject's unique characteristics. Orientation and thickness are determined as a function of features, such as subject weight, residual limb attributes, and activity level preferences (Michael 1987). Menard et al. advocates the Flex-Foot for people with amputation seeking active lifestyles. This is especially the case for those engaging in sports that include jumping (Menard et al. 1992). As implied, the Flex-Foot entails greater energy return characteristics relative to the Seattle Foot (Michael 1987; Menard et al. 1992). This observation is revealed by the fact that the Seattle Foot's energy storage and return assembly is constrained to the packaging of only the foot (Burgess et al. 1985).

By contrast the Flex-Foot's energy storage and return mechanism, which is comprised of graphite composite, utilizes a greater volume of the prosthetic foot and lower leg. This type of ankle-foot prosthesis spans the entire length from foot to the socket assembly. The design implication is the Flex-Foot is capable of storing and releasing energy throughout the prosthetic system, rather than being constrained to a four inch keel. This scheme facilitates responsiveness (Michael 1987).

The functional utility of the Flex-Foot is underscored by its successful applications in the context of active lifestyle endeavors. For example a volleyball player with amputation have commented on improving the ability to vertically leap. Other anecdotes involve the ability of a Flex-Foot user substantially improving the ability to complete a full marathon (Michael 1987). With its success the Flex-Foot is frequently recommended within the energy storage and return class of prosthesis (Hsu et al. 2006).

6.4 C-Walk

A more recent evolution within the energy storage and return prosthesis category is the 1C40 Otto Bock C-Walk. The C-Walk is slightly more mechanically complex as it consists of four primary supporting components:

- Carbon fiber reinforced plastic C-spring
- Carbon fiber reinforced plastic base spring
- Control ring with polymer insert
- Heel element

An advantage of the C-Walk is the claim that it facilitates an assortment of diverse activities, such as leisurely (slow) walking, faster walking speeds, and recreational activities (Hsu et al. 2006; Ottobock).

6.5 Testing and Evaluation of Energy Storage and Return Prostheses

Hsu et al. conducted a research study that contrasted energy storage and return prostheses, such as the Flex-Foot and C-Walk, to the more traditional solid ankle cushioned heel prosthesis. The investigation encompassed multiple roles for assessing physiologic aspects of gait, such as rating of perceived exertion, exercise intensity, energy expenditure, and gait efficiency, and pedometers to assess daily physical activity profiles. The researchers anticipated that the energy storage and return prostheses would yield superior parameters in terms of pedometer readings and physiological aspects relative to the solid ankle cushioned heel (Hsu et al. 2006).

The pedometer was worn throughout the day from morning (awake) to night (sleep). The subjects utilize the pedometer for all three prosthesis scenarios for the duration of 1 month each. The measurements from the pedometer were recorded in a logbook (Hsu et al. 2006).

The physiological parameters were acquired with the use of a treadmill. The treadmill aspect of the experiment incorporated multiple velocities relative to the self-selected walking velocity. Energy expenditure was derived as a function of oxygen consumption. Gait efficiency was based on oxygen consumption divided by speed. Relative exercise intensity was calculated as exercise heat rate per age predicted maximum heart rate. Rate of perceived exertion was based on the interpretation of a scale. The study incorporated a metabolic cart for evaluating oxygen consumption levels. The heart rate was acquired through radio-telemetry (Hsu et al. 2006).

In terms of pedometer data the trend favored the Flex-Foot for physical activity in terms of steps per day. The Flex-Foot and C-Walk provided generally lower energy expenditures tendencies in contrast to the solid ankle cushioned heel prosthesis. The C-Walk and Flex-Foot displayed reduced relative exercise intensity compared to the solid ankle cushioned heel prosthesis with the Flex-Foot attaining statistical significance. The C-Walk and Flex-Foot demonstrated better gait efficiency relative to the solid ankle cushioned heel prosthesis. The Flex-Foot enabled significantly reduced rate of perceived exertion compared to the C-Walk and solid ankle cushioned heel prosthesis. Overall the two energy storage and return prostheses (C-Walk and Flex-Foot) demonstrated improved performance when contrasted to the solid ankle cushioned heel prosthesis (Hsu et al. 2006).

Altering manufacturing techniques can modify performance of a specific type of energy storage and return prosthesis. Fey et al. investigated the effect of varying the stiffness of the prosthesis. Three levels of stiffness variation (compliant, nominal, and stiff) were achieved through an additive manufacturing technology. Modulating the stiffness of the prosthesis induced modifications in gait patterns for both the residual (prosthetic) limb and intact limb. The experimental gait analysis included EMG, force plates, and motion capture. With regards to the residual limb reducing prosthetic stiffness can increase range of motion and energy return during the mid to late aspects of stance phase. Notably, dorsiflexion about the residual limb displayed an increasing trend in proportion to decreasing the stiffness of the prosthesis. In summary, Fey et al. recommend that the degree of stiffness should be specified as a basis of subject specific mobility goals (Fey et al. 2011).

The nature of the energy storage and release type of prosthesis is functionally robust. However, the spring energy system is inherently limited. The principle of the conservation of energy implies that the energy released back into the gait cycle during terminal aspect of stance can never exceed a fraction of the energy stored upon initial contact during the preliminary phase of stance (Serway 1990; LeMoyne 2015).

Another issue that the energy storage and return class of prosthesis lacks the inherent timing features intrinsic to the ankle-foot complex. As implied in a previous Chap. 2: 'Ankle-foot complex and the fundamental aspects of gait' encompassing the considerable neurological influence of the ankle-foot complex a significant level of temporal regulation is implied regarding its activity during fluid and synchronous gait patterns. For example, the ankle-foot complex entails substantial effect from afferent and efferent neural pathways, which are further influenced by highly complex neurological structures, such as the central pattern generator and brain (Dobkin 2003; LeMoyne et al. 2008).

A solution of the topic of providing optimal temporal acuity with regards to energy release involves integrating mechanisms capable of controlling the timed release of elastic energy. Such an envisioned version of prosthesis would essentially consist of mechatronic devices capable of holding stored spring energy, while releasing the energy at the optimal aspect of stance phase.

6.6 Controlled Energy Storage and Return

Zelik envisioned a Controlled Energy Storage and Return (CESR) prosthesis. The progressive research development testing and evaluation of the CESR led to a Ph.D. dissertation for Dr. Zelik at the University of Michigan. The laboratory of Professor Kuo his Doctoral Committee Chair facilitated the research. The CESR prosthetic foot is comprised of a volumetric package that resembles of its predecessor the Seattle Foot. However the CESR is equipped with an assortment of supporting microelectronic derived components (Zelik 2012). The CESR constitutes a mechatronic evolution of the established energy storage and release prosthesis.

The functionality of the controlled energy storage and return prosthesis emphasized four aspects of stance phase. The design is intended to capture and release energy that is generally dissipated during the impact aspects of gait. The prosthesis is featured with a carbon fiber forefoot and heel assemblies. During the foot loading phase of stance energy is stored and locked through a one-way clutch. The potential energy level of the spring is sustained by the clutch mechanism during the mid-stance aspect of gait cycle. Additional energy is stored during the deflection of the carbon fiber forefoot (Collins and Kuo 2010; Zelik et al. 2011; Segal et al. 2012; Zelik 2012).

The timing of the energy release is controlled with the ability to augment the powered plantar flexion phase of terminal stance. A particular advantage of this prosthetic system is the capacity to modify the spring stiffness properties to the benefit of the patient. This configuration represents an advance regarding energy return relative to standard passive prostheses (Collins and Kuo 2010; Zelik et al. 2011; Segal et al. 2012; Zelik 2012).

The timing of the stored potential energy release is a function of the progressive loading of the forefoot assembly. Upon exceeding a load threshold based on the feedback of a force sensor positioned on the forefoot assembly, a clutch releases stored energy during the push-off phase of stance while the forefoot become progressively unloaded. The timed energy release is intended to emulate the temporal features of the standard ankle-foot complex during push-off. The controlled energy storage and return prosthesis is returned to a reset position during the swing phase by a small return spring (Collins and Kuo 2010).

This configuration stores and then releases energy through passive mechanisms in a robust manner. In order to control the energy storage and release active elements are incorporated. A microcontroller regulates the energy of the spring. Two micro-motors mechanically actuate the release of the energy storage spring and mechanism reset. The prosthesis requires about 0.8 W of power that is provided by a small battery (Collins and Kuo 2010).

The battery and microcontroller can be encased in a small backpack with a mass of approximately 0.8 kg. The microcontroller can attach to the prosthesis by ribbon cable. Analog data can be conveyed for acquisition through a coaxial cable (Zelik 2012). This prosthetic configuration entails substantially less battery power compared to state of the art electromechanical actuated powered prosthesis (LeMoyne 2015).

Conclusion

Advances regarding the development of technology for the domain of transtibial prostheses are highly correlated to the progression of scientific discovery for the understanding of the gait cycle. Until recent the design focus toward the development of prosthesis applications for people with transtibial amputation placed an emphasis on structural considerations. During the 1980s gait analysis elucidated a major finding that a substantial amount of mechanical power is provided to the gait cycle during the terminal aspect of stance phase known as powered plantar flexion. This discovery underscored the objective of providing energy about the terminal phase of stance through some means of energy return. Prior to the development of powered prostheses, prostheses with ability to store energy during preliminary stance phase with the release of energy upon reaching the terminal aspect of stance were developed. The ESAR class of prosthesis progressively evolved with applications incorporating elastic deflection about a keel encased in a prosthetic representative foot to applications that promote elastic deflection between the socket to the foot assembly of the prosthesis. The ESAR prosthesis constitutes a desirable alternative for people with amputation seeking highly active lifestyles. Although the ESAR prosthesis provides a functionally robust application, there is a lack of the ability to control the temporal release of the stored energy. With the assistance of mechatronic subsystems the Controlled Energy Storage and Return (CESR) demonstrated the ability to regulate the timing of the energy release. The CESR type of prosthesis is capable of achieving this objective through the use of a microelectronics package and clutch mechanism that controls the temporal release of the potential energy. These configurations of energy storage and return prostheses been thoroughly applied to testing and evaluation. Subject qualitative assessment and quantified gait analysis have underscored the benefits of these energy storage and return prostheses.

References

Burgess EM, Poggi DL, Hittenberger DA, Zettl JH, Moeller DE, Carpenter KL, Forsgren SM (1985) Development and preliminary evaluation of the VA Seattle foot. J Rehabil Res Dev 22:75–84

Collins SH, Kuo AD (2010) Recycling energy to restore impaired ankle function during human walking. PLoS One 5:e9307

Dobkin BH (2003) The clinical science of neurologic rehabilitation. Oxford University Press, New York

Fey NP, Klute GK, Neptune RR (2011) The influence of energy storage and return foot stiffness on walking mechanics and muscle activity in below-knee amputees. Clin Biomech 26:1025–1032

Hsu MJ, Nielsen DH, Lin-Chan SJ, Shurr D (2006) The effects of prosthetic foot design on physiologic measurements, self-selected walking velocity, and physical activity in people with transtibial amputation. Arch Phys Med Rehabil 87:123–129

LeMoyne R (2015) Advances regarding powered prosthesis for transtibial amputation. J Mech Med Biol 15:1–34

LeMoyne R, Coroian C, Mastroianni T, Grundfest W (2008) Virtual proprioception. J Mech Med Biol 8:317–338

Menard MR, McBride ME, Sanderson DJ, Murray DD (1992) Comparative biomechanical analysis of energy-storing prosthetic feet. Arch Phys Med Rehabil 73:451–458

Michael J (1987) Energy storing feet: a clinical comparison. Clin Prosthet Orthot 11:154–168

Ottobock. http://www.ottobock.com

Reswick JB (1986) Evaluation of the Seattle foot. J Rehabil Res Dev 23:77–94

Seattle foot. http://prosthetics.umwblogs.org/the-seattle-foot/

Segal AD, Zelik KE, Klute GK, Morgenroth DC, Hahn ME, Orendurff MS, Adamczyk PG, Collins SH, Kuo AD, Czerniecki JM (2012) The effects of a controlled energy storage and return prototype prosthetic foot on transtibial amputee ambulation. Hum Mov Sci 31:918–931

Serway RA (1990) Physics for scientists and engineers. Saunders College, Philadelphia

Zelik KE (2012) Passive energy-saving mechanisms in human locomotion. Ph.D. dissertation, University of Michigan, Department of Mechanical Engineering, Ann Arbor

Zelik KE, Collins SH, Adamczyk PG, Segal AD, Klute GK, Morgenroth DC, Hahn ME, Orendurff MS, Czerniecki JM, Kuo AD (2011) Systematic variation of prosthetic foot spring affects center-of-mass mechanics and metabolic cost during walking. IEEE Trans Neural Syst Rehabil Eng 19:411–419

Chapter 7
Architecture of a Powered Prosthesis System: Actuators, Sensors, and Control

Abstract A current strategy for providing a powered prosthesis capable of emulating the intricate features of the ankle-foot complex is through the application of the robotic architecture. The proposed robotic architecture consists of three levels: actuators, sensors, and control. An emphasis is placed upon the actuator level, for which the series elastic actuator is a subject of prosthetic research and development, and other types of actuators, such as the chemical-derived actuator and pneumatic actuator. Inclusive of the subject of actuators are advanced concepts that extend the technology of the series elastic actuator, such as the Robotic Tendon, with variable stiffness. A new perspective on muscle modeling that accommodates history dependence is featured, which is known as the Winding Filament Hypothesis. As a supplement, battery technology is discussed with a consideration of future capability. The sensor level addresses currently applied microelectronic devices, such as accelerometers, gyroscopes, angular encoders, linear encoders, and footswitches. The control level focuses on the application of the finite state machine, which derives the status of gait based on the acuity of sensor feedback.

Keywords Robotic architecture • Actuator level • Series elastic actuator • Sensor level • Control level

7.1 Introduction

A powered prosthesis constitutes a robust robotic system that utilizes the perspective of a robotic architecture. A robotic architecture can encompass a system that utilizes the following general aspects:

- Actuators
- Sensors
- Control

The actuator level imparts mechanical interaction with the environment, such as powered plantar flexion during the gait cycle. The control level regulates the interaction of the actuator level. The decision process of the control level is based on data acquired from the sensor level (Brooks 1986; Bekey 2005; LeMoyne 2015).

R. LeMoyne, *Advances for Prosthetic Technology*,
DOI 10.1007/978-4-431-55816-3_7

The robotic architecture of a powered prosthesis represents an analogy to the human ankle-foot complex discussed in the previous Chap. 2: 'Ankle-foot complex and the fundamental aspects of gait'. The actuator can be considered similar in objective to human musculature. The sensor level can be compared relative to proprioception and cutaneous afferent input. Neurology, such as the central pattern generator and motor cortex, are analogous to the control level of a robotic system.

The goal of this chapter is to provide a broad coverage of these integral aspects of a robotic architecture. An emphasis is placed on the actuator level. This topic regarding robotic architecture for the scope of the powered prosthesis is a continual subject of research and academic contribution that is still a subject of debate.

7.2 Actuator Level, Imparting Mechanical Energy for the Powered Prosthesis

In the case of a powered prosthesis the actuator principally provides mechanical energy to the gait cycle, such as through powered plantar flexion (Bekey 2005; LeMoyne 2015). The utility of a particular type of actuator is its power to weight ratio and the energy density of its energy source (Bekey 2005; Paine 2014).

For the scope of this chapter various types of actuators are discussed regarding their context for powered actuation of a transtibial prosthesis:

- Chemical-derived actuator
- Pneumatic actuator
- Series elastic actuator
- Robotic Tendon
- Winding Filament Hypothesis; an advanced biomimetic actuator concept

The topic of the battery is included, since it constitutes the electrical energy source for electromechanical actuators.

7.2.1 Chemical-Derived Actuator

The concept of the chemical actuator is derived from established rocket propulsion technology. Fundamental to the application is the use of a hypergolic propellant. A propellant that is hypergolic undergoes energy producing (exothermic) combustion upon contact with a substrate. Hydrogen peroxide for example has a hypergolic reaction with silver (Sutton 1992).

The hypergolic combustion of hydrogen peroxide yields water, oxygen, and considerable energy. In a closed volume scenario, the byproducts can be expanded in the context of a gas generator. This application can be utilized to impart mechanical energy for an actuator (Goldfarb et al. 2003).

A monopropellant derived actuator developed by Goldfarb et al. has been realized. The decomposition of hydrogen peroxide pressurizes a hot gas reservoir. The hydrogen peroxide tank is pressurized by an inert gas and regulated through a valve to the control the extent of the exothermic reaction. The hot gas reservoir products (water as steam and oxygen) are controlled through a 4-way proportional valve to the gas actuator section, which provides the mechanical actuation. With their energy content reduced by providing mechanical energy the hot gasses are then expelled into the ambient atmosphere (Goldfarb et al. 2003).

Chemical combustion, such as through a hypergolic monopropellant, offers attractive energy density characteristics. This configuration offers roughly an order of magnitude advance in actuation potential relative to conventional DC battery powered actuators. The proposed actuator consists of an aggregate mass of 1.5 kg. A 70 % hydrogen peroxide solution was applied. The exhaust exceeds a temperature threshold of 100 C (Goldfarb et al. 2003).

Although this monopropellant actuator configuration offers considerable utility from the scope of a performance perspective, there are multiple issues for the integration of the actuator within the context of a human user interface. Hydrogen peroxide even when diluted, but capable of hypergolic combustion, is considered highly toxic from an environmental perspective. Even in the domain of rocket propulsion hydrogen peroxide is currently seldom used (Sutton 1992).

Another issue of concern is the robust storage and even refilling requirements. Furthermore, the considerable temperature of the byproducts constitutes a hazard to the user and surrounding environment. With a heat source exceeding 100 C, the potential for thermal soak throughout the prosthesis would be preclusive.

7.2.2 *Pnuematic Actuator*

During the later 1950s McKibben developed a pneumatic actuator system for providing orthotic assistance for people with polio (Nickel et al. 1963; Klute et al. 2000). The actuator utilized pneumatics (compressed air) as its energy source. A rubber bladder was sheathed with a helical weave consisting of nylon. Upon inflation the McKibben actuator would contract, exhibiting muscle like features on activation (Gaylord 1958; Klute et al. 2000; Bekey 2005).

Klute et al. proposed the McKibben actuator as suitable for the muscle like actuation of a transtibial prosthesis. The application by Klute et al. integrates a series spring and parallel hydraulic damper in tandem with the McKibben actuator for exhibiting muscle-like qualities. Experimental test and evaluation demonstrates properties that are comparable to muscle like actuation (Klute et al. 2000). One notable issue with this type of pneumatic actuator configuration is the requirement for a compressed air source, such as a pneumatic line or a compressed air tank (Bekey 2005; LeMoyne 2015).

However, the pneumatic actuator configuration for a powered prosthesis warrants further consideration. This type of actuator constitutes a highly cost effective scheme as the medium for the energy source is compressed air. Although, generally precluded from an autonomous environment, the pneumatic actuator may be highly useful in a clinical rehabilitation setting.

For example, consider a military rehabilitation setting. A veteran is in the process of undergoing rehabilitation from a recent amputation. With regards to the phased rehabilitation transition to ambulatory walking with a powered prosthesis, a cost-effective pneumatic actuator powered prosthesis may provide a useful increment during the rehabilitation process.

7.2.3 Series Elastic Actuator

The series elastic actuator is the most prevalent type of actuator incorporated into lower limb powered prostheses. The primary components to the series elastic actuator are a DC motor that is aligned in series with a spring. As the actuator requires a source of electric energy, a battery is generally included with the application (Cherelle et al. 2014; Grimmer and Seyfarth 2014; LeMoyne 2015). The series elastic actuator constitutes a substantial paradigm shift in robotic technology.

Prior to the innovation of the series elastic actuator, the overriding perspective with respect to actuator selection was oriented toward maximal stiffness. This perspective was based on the assumption that increasing actuator stiffness enables optimal position control bandwidth, stability, and precision. In general, an actuator that provides considerable stiffness about the interface attenuates position errors for a respective load environment (Pratt and Williamson 1995).

However, the traditional design standpoint for pursuing increased stiffness entails multiple negative consequences. Because of the torque density characteristics of electromechanical actuators, a gearing assembly is frequently incorporated. However, the traditional actuator is susceptible to failure modes with associated gearing, such as noise, friction, and ripple of torque loads. Sensitivity to torque load constitutes a concern for the robustness of the application. Reflected inertia and friction about the gear trains can be a source of environmental damage with regards to the actuator (Pratt and Williamson 1995).

The contextual environment for a suitable actuator subsystem to support a robust powered prosthesis should be emphasized. Intuitively, walking constitutes a highly variable and somewhat unpredictable environment. An actuator assembly that function in such a scenario would be desirable. An actuator subsystem that enables an energy efficient and biomimetic equivalent to the highly intricate musculotendon features of the intact ankle-foot complex as revealed in a previous Chap. 2: 'Ankle-foot complex and the fundamental aspects of gait' constitutes a design objective. The inclusion of control capabilities at the actuator level would permit a simplified architecture more representative of the autonomy of natural walking.

During the mid 1990s Pratt and Williamson of MIT developed a revolutionary actuator that has since its establishment has become a ubiquitous aspect of most modern powered prostheses that incorporate an electro-mechanical actuator. The design is more biologically similar to the synergistic capabilities of the muscle and tendon. The series elastic actuator consists of three major aspects:

- motor
- gear train
- series elasticity

Series elasticity can be provided by a spring that interacts between the load and gear train with motor (Pratt and Williamson 1995).

One of the benefits to an innovation at the actuator level is that other levels of robotic architecture can benefit. The inclusion of an eloquent and more biologically representative actuator level can augment and complement more complex levels, such as the control level (Bekey 2005). The advance of the series elastic actuator exemplifies the synergistic interaction between the supporting subsystems, such as an actuator, and global systems, such as a biomimetic powered prosthesis (LeMoyne 2015).

The advance of the series elastic actuator constitutes multiple benefits to the actuator technology space. Three of these benefits are:

- Low pass shock filtering
- Enhanced force control
- Augmented energy storage

In summary these utilities are effectively obscured from the higher level control system (Pratt and Williamson 1995). The series elastic actuator can possibly also benefit the control level by reducing software complexity. Other design constrains, such as real-time processing of software, processor speed, and battery requirements, are likely alleviated.

The positioning of a spring assembly adjacent to the gearing assembly enables a low pass filter with regards to shock loads imparted on the actuator. By attenuating shock loads, the peak forces on the gearing are considerably reduced. The enhanced elasticity augments the actuator's robustness to shock tolerance (Pratt and Williamson 1995). The incorporation of shock tolerance about the actuator level can potentially improve the evolutionary outlook for the powered prosthesis technology space.

The typical activity level for a person entails on the order of 1000s of steps a day (Herr and Grabowski 2012; LeMoyne 2015). A robust actuator should satisfy a user's activity level. Also, a well designed powered prosthesis should satisfy as protracted a design life cycle as feasible. Therefore, an actuator that incorporates a means to ameliorate shock loads, which are an inherent aspect of typical walking, would constitute an appealing inclusion into the actuator level of the powered prosthesis.

The integration of series elasticity for an actuator benefits the control level. Essentially the series elastic actuator reduces the issue of force control to a topic of position control. The displacement of the series spring is resultant of a specific force load from a known spring constant. Therefore, output force is directly proportional to spring displacement. Position is considered more simple to control with regards to a gear train than force control. This technique of deriving force control on the basis of position control reduced force error, thereby advancing the acuity of force accuracy (Pratt and Williamson 1995).

The improvement in an actuator's capacity to accurately determine force can positively benefit the control level architecture. Advancing force accuracy can likely reduce software complexity for a closed feedback loop for ascertaining the true force output. As the powered prosthesis is a synergistically packaged device, constraints in terms of software complexity in a real-time context, processor speed, and battery requirements may be alleviated.

Incorporating series elasticity into an actuator design facilitates the capacity to store energy. In the context of an actuator for locomotion, energy storage can substantially improve efficiency (Pratt and Williamson 1995). Including the capability to store energy within an actuator constitutes a major advance for the objective of developing biomimetic actuators. During human locomotion musculature and associated tendons enable the ability to elastically store and release energy in a biologically advantageous method (Ishikawa et al. 2005).

Improvements with respect to the conservation of energy have broad implications for the powered prosthesis. Battery requirements can be reduced. With the actuator force output requirements relaxed, due to available stored energy, the life cycle of the actuator can be advanced. The total number of steps for a full battery charge may be increased.

The placement of an elastic element relative to the associated actuator permits multifunctional capabilities that provide utility to a variety of activity levels. The elastic actuator currently has been identified with multiple elastic elements. For example an elastic element may be oriented in series or parallel relative to the actuator, which represents the contractile element (Grimmer and Seyfarth 2014).

Grimmer and Seyfarth have identified 11 configurations that compliment the innovation of the series elastic actuator. These configurations consist of various placements of series and parallel elements relative to the actuator. Alternative strategies incorporate unidirectional springs that engage only for specified movement pathways, a clutching mechanism to regulate motion, and damping elements placed either in series or parallel orientation (Grimmer and Seyfarth 2014).

The strategic and predetermined placement of an energy conserving element, such as a spring, has been demonstrated in the context of research and development for alleviating design constraints relative to the actuator. The research of Dr. Herr's laboratory at MIT amended a parallel spring to their powered prosthesis, which substantially reduced load requirements for the series elastic actuator (Au et al. 2007; Au 2007; Au and Herr 2008; LeMoyne 2015).

The presence of a parallel spring accommodates the powered prosthetic by greatly reducing the force requirements on the series elastic actuator and improved force bandwidth characteristics (Au et al. 2007; Au and Herr 2008). Force bandwidth is essential to the robust design of actuator. The force bandwidth is a parameter that signifies the responsiveness of the actuator based on a prescribed force setting (Robinson 2000). Other powered prosthesis applications have reduced their actuator power requirements by over a factor of two with the proper placement of its elastic element (Grimmer and Seyfarth 2014).

7.2.4 Robotic Tendon

The Robotic Tendon represents a progressive evolution of the series actuator concept. The strategic selection of the spring configuration greatly influences the performance characteristics of the overall series elastic actuator (Au et al. 2007; Au and Herr 2008; LeMoyne 2015). Intuitively, an actuator design that is capable of varying its elasticity as a function of use context would be highly desirable. Hollander et al. have developed a Robotic Tendon that possesses such adjustable qualities (Hollander et al. 2005).

The Robotic Tendon actuator features a spring assembly that can adjust the number of active spring coils that facilitate the actuator, which is denoted as a Jack Spring. By adjusting the quantity of active coils the spring stiffness is modulated. For this integrated configuration both energy storage and compliance facilitate the actuator objectives (Hollander et al. 2005).

The Robotic Tendon resembles the biomimetic attributes of human musculature, especially regarding intrinsic elasticity. With the incorporation of such elastic properties, the peak power and work requirements of the actuator can be reduced. Therefore the electric motor can be downscaled to decrease weight, which imparts considerable benefit to the entire quality of the powered prosthesis (Hollander et al. 2005).

In order to quantify the benefits of the Robotic Tendon actuator, preliminary analysis was applied to a 80 kg representative subject. The walking rate was 0.8Hz. This scenario establishes a peak power requirement of 250 W. For the direct drive contingency, a 250 W continuous power motor, such as a Maxon RE75, would be required. The aggregate mass of the motor (2.8 kg) and gearbox (3.8 kg) would be approximately 6.6 kg, which would be highly cumbersome for a transtibial prosthesis application (Hollander et al. 2005).

The Robotic Tendon actuator would be capable of providing a peak power of 250 W, but would only require a 90 W motor, such as the Maxon RE35, which only has a mass of 0.34 kg. The entire Robotic Tendon actuator assembly has been estimated to has a mass of 0.84 kg. This actuator configuration with adjustable stiffness represents approximately an eightfold mass savings relative to the conventional design (Hollander et al. 2005).

7.2.5 *The Winding Filament Hypothesis, an Advanced Biomimetic Actuator Concept*

The primary objective of the technology evolution of advanced prostheses is to develop systems that are as biomimetic as possible. Attempts have been made to incorporate neuromuscular models into the control architecture. Markowitz et al. and Eilenberg et al. achieved this ambition through the incorporation of the Hill model (Eilenberg et al. 2010; Markowitz et al. 2011).

The Hill model is a widely accepted and standard muscle model that was originally developed during the 1930s. The muscle model is the prevailing strategy for estimating the force production as a consequence of muscle activation (Hill 1938; Bekey 2005). The Winding Filament Hypothesis constitutes a paradigm shift with regards to muscle modeling as it better accounts for muscle history dependence. Phenomena, such as force enhancement and force depression, are more appropriately demonstrated through the Winding Filament Hypothesis (Nishikawa et al. 2012, 2013). However, before describing the conceptual perspective of the Winding Filament Hypothesis, an elucidation of the evolutionary trends that facilitated the understanding of muscle modeling is warranted.

Muscle modeling has progressively evolved over the course of the past century. The synthesis of muscle modeling into a more cohesive and biomimetic description has been the integral consequence of scientific discovery and engineering/mathematical modeling and analysis. During the 1930s Hill envisioned a model for characterizing muscle activity with the emphasis on contractile and elastic elements (Hill 1938; Bekey 2005). Then in the 1950s Huxley proposed the sliding filament model, which was widely accepted and serves as a ubiquitous aspect of standard textbooks that are academically distributed. The essence of the sliding filament model is that force production is developed through actin myofilaments sliding over myosin myofilaments (Kandel et al. 2000; Seeley et al. 2003). Later in the 1980s Zajac advanced the Hill model with a better characterization of the muscle tendon relationship (Zajac 1989). Currently, the Zajac model is incorporated in well-accepted computational muscle modeling programs, such as OpenSim (Thelen 2003; Opensim).

The role and even the discovery of titin did not occur in arrangement with the progressive evolution and acceptance of the Hill model and sliding filament model (Nishikawa et al. 2012, 2013; LeMoyne 2015). Titin was actually discovered during the decade of the 1970s, which is on the order of two decades after the establishment of the sliding filament model and four decades subsequent to the Hill model (Maruyama 1976; Wang et al. 1979; Nishikawa et al. 2012). The role of titin for muscle behavior serves a critical purpose for the subject of the topic of muscle history dependence (Nishikawa et al. 2012, 2013).

Until recent, the subject muscle history dependence, such as force depression and force enhancement, was not considered a significant aspect for modeling muscle force production. Conventional muscle models generally do not account for the role of muscle history dependence. In consideration of the correlated isometric force production estimations imply that force enhancement and force depression can attain 50 % greater and lesser force production, respective. The quest for higher fidelity muscle modeling that accounts for history dependence has become a subject of mounting interest (Herzog 2004).

History dependent muscle models, which are phenomenological and empirical in concept, can be developed (Forcinito et al. 1998; Ettema and Meijer 2000; Ettema 2002). Forcinito et al. developed a strategy for estimating force enhancement and force depression attributes through incorporating a contractile element, linear spring, linear dashpot, and elastic rack. The elastic rack engages with activation (Forcinito et al. 1998). Ettema and Meijer contrasted a Hill model with modifications to account for muscle contractile history with model incorporating exponential decay to emulate the mechno-chemistry of the cross bridge cycle, using empirically determined parameters (Ettema and Meijer 2000). Ettema compared the conventional Hill model to a modified Hill model that accommodates history effects. These disparate models were contrasted to the scope of a joint system incorporating agonist/antagonist musculature. The findings reveal that the augmented Hill model which addresses muscle history enables relatively better stability attributes compared to the conventional Hill model (Ettema 2002).

In stark contrast to the highly phenomenological and empirical history dependent muscle modeling perspectives is the Winding Filament Hypothesis. The Winding Filament Hypothesis effectively evolves the sliding filament model with the consideration of titin. Note that titin was discovered on the order of two decades following the establishment of Huxley's sliding filament model. Titin serves the subject of muscle force production respective of two domains: neuromuscular and potential energy storage. The neuromuscular role of titin is based on the N2A region of titin binding to the thin actin filament from the release of Ca^{2+} from the action potential of an efferent neuron. Titin interacts with the thin actin filament through linear translation and winding rotation with the elastic PEVK segment of titin retaining potential energy. Force enhancement and force depression aspects of muscle history dependence are accounted for in the biologically cohesive Winding Filament Hypothesis (Nishikawa et al. 2012, 2013; Tester et al. 2012; Yeo 2012).

A mechanistic analog of the Winding Filament Hypothesis has been developed, and the optimization of the model is a topic of current research. General renditions of the model entail the following aspects. A pulley simulates the mechanical equivalence of titin N2A binding to the thin actin filament with associated rotation. On one aspect of the pulley resides a contractile element in parallel with a viscous damper, and the other aspect resides a titin representative spring. When the contractile element is activated a torque balance is achieved. The center of the pulley is mounted to a series spring (Tester et al. 2012; Petak et al. 2013a, b). The efficacy of the Winding Filament Hypothesis is currently being evaluated regarding applications for an actuator and as a software platform for a powered prosthesis (Nishikawa and Uyeno 2010; LeMoyne et al. 2013, 2014a; Petak 2014).

A particularly interesting aspect of the Winding Filament Hypothesis is in consideration to control architecture and neurological plasticity. The temporal sensitivity of muscle history dependence has been noted as brisker relative to the neurological reflex loop (Nichols and Houk 1976; Nishikawa et al. 2012, 2013). The implication is that an actuator incorporating the Winding Filament Hypothesis may advance the quality of the control architecture from the actuator level. Also the quality of neuro-adaptation, such as plasticity, for the user of a Winding Filament Hypothesis type actuator may be augmented, which would benefit people with amputation utilizing a powered prosthesis that incorporates the Winding Filament Hypothesis.

7.2.6 Battery

All actuators require a stored energy source to convert the respective potential energy to actuator resultant mechanical energy (Grimmer and Seyfarth 2014). For the chemical derived actuator developed by Goldfarb et al. a storable monopropellant, such as concentrated hydrogen peroxide, was used (Goldfarb et al. 2003). For pneumatic actuators applied by Klute et al. a tethered source of compressed air through a line enabled the energy source (Klute et al. 2000). The most prevalent actuator and energy source combination is the electromechanical actuator that utilizes a battery as its energy source (Grimmer and Seyfarth 2014).

The lithium-ion and lithium-ion polymer battery have been applied to the powered transtibial prosthetic domain (Grimmer and Seyfarth 2014). The concept of the lithium ion battery is based on the mobility of the lithium ion during both discharge and charge status. The lithium ion battery offers a superior energy density relative to other conventional batteries, such as the nickel-cadmium type battery (Panasonic). During the 1990s Sony Corporation introduced the first commercial application involving the lithium-ion battery. The lithium-ion battery facilitates substantial advances in the consumer electronic industry, which likely will promote correlated evolution for devices, such as powered prosthetics (Economist).

A further evolution of the lithium-ion type of battery is the lithium-ion polymer battery. The primary unique design feature of the lithium-ion polymer is the use of a solid polymer electrolyte. The advantage is the lithium-ion polymer battery can be shaped according to the volumetric packaging constraints of the application, such as a mobile phone, computer notebook, or especially the packaging requirements of a powered prosthesis (Stephan and Nahm 2006).

As the battery constitutes an aspect of considerable impact for the consumer electronics industry, substantial research and development endeavors will likely yield more associated breakthrough technologies. A future advance within the scope of battery technology is the lithium-air battery. A lithium-air battery constitutes a considerable shift from current battery configurations. At the anode the lithium undergoes electrochemical oxidation. Air from the ambient surrounding provides oxygen for reduction at the cathode. The lithium-air battery offers an energy density on the scale of gasoline at approximately 1700 Wh/kg, which is approximately ten times greater than the Li-ion battery (160 Wh/kg) and 40 times more than the conventional nickel-cadmium battery (40 Wh/kg) (Girishkumar et al. 2010).

Overall, commercial electronic demands are envisioned to induce considerable evolutionary trends for the battery, respective of applied research and development. The anticipated effect for the domain of the powered prostheses would be significant improvements in terms of mass reduction, volumetric packaging, and operational usage.

7.3 Sensor Level, Perceptivity of the Powered Prosthesis Status During Gait Cycle

For a robotic powered prosthesis, the sensors constitute the afferent perceptivity of the device. A previous Chap. 2: 'Ankle-foot complex and the fundamental aspects of gait' underscores the role of sensory feedback to neural structures, such as the central pattern generator and brain. Sensor components provide status feedback for the control system architecture of the powered prosthesis.

There are five primary types of sensors employed for the majority of powered prostheses. These sensors provide feedback acuity regarding the spatial representation of the global prosthesis, the activity status of moving assemblies, such as the ankle joint and actuator, and degree of interaction with ground contact. The most prevalent sensors are:

- Accelerometers
- Gyroscopes
- Angular encoders
- Linear encoders
- Footswitches (Grimmer and Seyfarth 2014)

Accelerometers and gyroscopes provide feedback regarding the spatial representation of the sensor location. Both are currently implemented as microelectronic devices, and they are readily applied to highly ubiquitous applications, such as smartphones. These sensors are trending toward further miniaturization, as many industries are benefiting from their research and development. The accelerometer measures acceleration, and the gyroscope measures the rate of angular rotation (LeMoyne et al. 2008, 2009, 2014b; LeMoyne and Mastroianni 2014, 2015).

The encoder is designed to measure displacement in a linear or angular direction. In general for a powered prosthesis, the encoder is positioned about the ankle joint to determine rotational status and also at the actuator to ascertain its level of activity (Bekey 2005; Grimmer and Seyfarth 2014). Two types of rotary encoders are the optical and magnetic encoder. The optical encoder operates with a light emitting diode that is incident on a photo-detector, with a series of slots on a disk. The magnetic encoder utilizes the Hall-effect to derive a signal through a disk's magnetic interaction with the Hall-effect sensor (Eitel 2014). Linear encoders determine linear displacement, and they can operate through similar conceptual principles, such as through optical or magnetic techniques (Nyce 2004).

The footswitch is a conventional gait analysis tool that measures the relationship of foot contact to the ground surface. This device can be readily applied to the powered prosthetic domain. With the strategic positioning of the multiple footswitches, the status of the prosthesis' relation to ground contact can be ascertained, which can provide the control system architecture acuity as to various transitional states (LeMoyne et al. 2008; LeMoyne 2015).

7.4 Control Level, Intelligent Assessment of the Powered Prosthesis Status During Gait Cycle

As the series elastic actuator provides a more biomimetic representation compared to previous devices for developing motive power, a similarly biomimetic control architecture should be developed. A major aspect of neurological regulation for human gait is the central pattern generator. The central pattern generator greatly facilitates the movement patterns with descending supraspinal command from the brain, such as the motor cortex. Such neurological structures critically rely on the afferent feedback. In particular proprioception represents a body's spatial perceptivity through muscle spindle afferents (Dietz 2002; Nolte and Sundsten 2002; Bekey 2005; Watson et al. 2010).

The development of an appropriate control level architecture constitutes a unique challenge in consideration of the design constraints. A standard PC may be capable of reducing data for a complex central pattern generator emulation. However for a battery constrained and geometrically constrained powered prosthesis, the control architecture must be reliable in a truly real-time environment. Also the software should be amenable to the processing time constraint implied by the computational capabilities of the powered prosthesis (Grimmer and Seyfarth 2014; LeMoyne 2015).

Furthermore, the sensor level should provide sufficient acuity to the control level. Too many sensors may encumber the mass, volume, and power constraints of a robust powered prosthesis. The relevance of the sensor package for feedback in terms of appropriateness and fidelity is also an advised subject of consideration (LeMoyne et al. 2011; LeMoyne 2015).

A well tested and evaluated control architecture that satisfies the qualities of neurological representation of gait is the finite state machine. The refinement of the finite state controller in the context of representing the phases and subphases of gait has been a subject of considerable research and development over the span of roughly four decades. During the 1970s Grimes proposed this type of control architecture for the application to a transfemoral prosthesis. The concept incorporates a finite state intent recognizer for identifying the appropriate phase transition of gait. Upon recognition the appropriate control architecture is applied (Grimes

1979). The finite state machine in principle identifies a respective state based on a series of contextually relevant threshold bounds. The phase state is established based on the feedback from pertinent sensors (Zlatnik et al. 2002; Bekey 2005; Au 2007; Au et al. 2008).

Conclusion
A synergistic perspective of the powered prosthesis is provided through the scheme of a three level robotic architecture. These three levels of the robotic architecture address the roles of mechanical actuation, sensory feedback, and intelligent control. Multiple actuator configurations of actuators are encompassed, such as chemical-derived, pneumatic, and series elastic actuators. Actuators with series elasticity demonstrate considerable promise in autonomous settings. An advanced concept, such as the Robotic Tendon, that enables variable stiffness is addressed. The Winding Filament Hypothesis is discussed as a novel muscle model that provides a biologically representative explanation of muscle history dependence. The battery constitutes a correlated technology for electro-mechanical actuators, and the current and future capabilities are addressed. Sensory level microelectronic devices, such as accelerometers, gyroscopes, angular encoders, linear encoders, and footswitches, provide feedback for the control level. The control level acquires the status of gait through applications, such as the finite state machine. The objective is to develop an integral approach for powered prostheses that enables an optimal biomimetic representation of the ankle-foot complex for people with transtibial amputation.

References

Au SK (2007) Powered ankle-foot prosthesis for the improvement of amputee walking economy. Ph.D. dissertation, MIT, Department of Mechanical Engineering, Cambridge

Au SK, Herr HM (2008) Powered ankle-foot prosthesis. IEEE Robot Autom Mag 15:52–59

Au SK, Herr H, Weber J, Martinez-Villalpando EC (2007) Powered ankle-foot prosthesis for the improvement of amputee ambulation. Proceedings of 29th annual international conference IEEE EMBS, Lyon, pp 3020–3026

Au S, Berniker M, Herr H (2008) Powered ankle-foot prosthesis to assist level-ground and stair-descent gaits. Neural Netw 21:654–666

Bekey GA (2005) Autonomous robots: from biological inspiration to implementation and control. MIT Press, Cambridge

Brooks R (1986) A robust layered control system for a mobile robot. IEEE J Robot Autom 2:14–23

Cherelle P, Mathijssen G, Wang Q, Vanderborght B, Lefeber D (2014) Advances in propulsive bionic feet and their actuation principles. Adv Mech Eng 6:1–21

Dietz V (2002) Proprioception and locomotor disorders. Nat Rev Neurosci 3:781–790

Economist. http://www.economist.com/node/1176209 (Technology Quarterly: Q2 2002 CASE HISTORY Hooked on lithium)

Eilenberg MF, Geyer H, Herr H (2010) Control of a powered ankle–foot prosthesis based on a neuromuscular model. IEEE Trans Neural Syst Rehabil Eng 18:164–173

Eitel E (2014) Basics of rotary encoders: overview and new technologies. Machine Design. http://machinedesign.com/sensors/basics-rotary-encoders-overview-and-new-technologies-0
Ettema GJ (2002) Effects of contraction history on control and stability in explosive actions. J Electromyogr Kinesiol 12:455–461
Ettema GJ, Meijer K (2000) Muscle contraction history: modified Hill versus an exponential decay model. Biol Cybern 83:491–500
Forcinito M, Epstein M, Herzog W (1998) Can a rheological muscle model predict force depression/enhancement? J Biomech 31:1093–1099
Gaylord RH (1958) Fluid actuated motor system and stroking device. U.S. Patent No. 2,844,126. U.S. Patent and Trademark Office, Washington, DC
Girishkumar G, McCloskey B, Luntz AC, Swanson S, Wilcke W (2010) Lithium – air battery: promise and challenges. J Phys Chem Lett 1:2193–2203
Goldfarb M, Barth EJ, Gogola M, Wehrmeyer J (2003) Design and energetic characterization of a liquid-propellant-powered actuator for self-powered robots. IEEE/ASME Trans Mechatron 8:254–262
Grimes DL (1979) An active multi-mode above-knee prosthesis controller. Ph.D. dissertation, MIT, Department of Mechanical Engineering, Cambridge
Grimmer M, Seyfarth A (2014) Mimicking human-like leg function in prosthetic limbs, chap 5. In: Artemiadis P (ed) Neuro-robotics: from brain machine interfaces to rehabilitation robotics. Springer, Dordrecht
Herr HM, Grabowski AM (2012) Bionic ankle–foot prosthesis normalizes walking gait for persons with leg amputation. Proc Biol Sci 279:457–464
Herzog W (2004) History dependence of skeletal muscle force production: implications for movement control. Hum Mov Sci 23:591–604
Hill AV (1938) The heat of shortening and the dynamic constants of muscle. Proc R Soc London B Biol Sci 126:136–195
Hollander KW, Sugar TG, Herring DE (2005) Adjustable Robotic Tendon using a 'Jack Spring'™. Proceedings of 9th international conference on rehabilitation robotics (ICORR 2005), Chicago, pp 113–118
Ishikawa M, Komi PV, Grey MJ, Lepola V, Bruggemann GP (2005) Muscle-tendon interaction and elastic energy usage in human walking. J Appl Physiol 99:603–608
Kandel ER, Schwartz JH, Jessell TM (2000) Principles of neural science. McGraw-Hill, New York
Klute GK, Czerniecki JM, Hannaford B (2000) Muscle-like pneumatic actuators for below-knee prostheses. Proceedings the 7th international conference on new actuators. Bremen, pp 289–292
LeMoyne R (2015) Advances regarding powered prosthesis for transtibial amputation. J Mech Med Biol 15:1–34
LeMoyne R, Mastroianni T (2014) Implementation of a smartphone as a wireless gyroscope application for the quantification of reflex response. Proceedings of 36th annual international conference IEEE EMBS, Chicago, pp 3654–3657
LeMoyne R, Mastroianni T (2015) Use of smartphones and portable media devices for quantifying human movement characteristics of gait, tendon reflex response, and Parkinson's disease hand tremor, chap 23. In: Rasooly A, Herold KE (eds) Mobile health technologies: methods and protocols. Springer, New York
LeMoyne R, Coroian C, Mastroianni T, Grundfest W (2008) Accelerometers for quantification of gait and movement disorders: a perspective review. J Mech Med Biol 8:137–152
LeMoyne R, Coroian C, Mastroianni T, Opalinski P, Cozza M, Grundfest W (2009) The merits of artificial proprioception, with applications in biofeedback gait rehabilitation concepts and movement disorder characterization, chap 10. In: Barros de Mello CA (ed) Biomedical engineering. Intech, Vienna
LeMoyne R, Mastroianni T, Coroian C, Grundfest W (2011) Tendon reflex and strategies for quantification, with novel methods incorporating wireless accelerometer reflex quantification devices, a perspective review. J Mech Med Biol 11:471–513

LeMoyne R, Nishikawa K, Tester J, Wilkinson K (2013) Winding filament model for remote robotic manipulation, NAU invention disclosure: 2013–015
LeMoyne R, Nishikawa K, Tester J, Hessel A (2014a) Ankle rehabilitation system using bioinspired muscle-like actuator, NAU invention disclosure: 2014–004
LeMoyne R, Mastroianni T, Montoya K (2014b) Implementation of a smartphone for evaluating gait characteristics of a trans-tibial prosthesis. Proceedings of 36th annual international conference IEEE EMBS, Chicago, pp 3674–3677
Markowitz J, Krishnaswamy P, Eilenberg MF, Endo K, Barnhart C, Herr H (2011) Speed adaptation in a powered transtibial prosthesis controlled with a neuromuscular model. Philos Trans R Soc Lond B Biol Sci 366:1621–1631
Maruyama K (1976) Connectin, an elastic protein from myofibrils. J Biochem 80:405–407
Nichols TR, Houk JC (1976) Improvement in linearity and regulation of stiffness that results from actions of stretch reflex. J Neurophysiol 39:119–142
Nickel VL, Perry J, Garrett AL (1963) Development of useful function in the severely paralyzed hand. J Bone Joint Surg 45:933–952
Nishikawa K, Uyeno TA (2010) Elastic motor-spring actuator. U.S. Patent Application 13/203,185
Nishikawa KC, Monroy JA, Uyeno TE, Yeo SH, Pai DK, Lindstedt SL (2012) Is titin a 'winding filament'? A new twist on muscle contraction. Proc Biol Sci 279:981–990
Nishikawa KC, Monroy JA, Powers KL, Gilmore LA, Uyeno TA, Lindstedt SL (2013) A molecular basis for intrinsic muscle properties: implications for motor control, chap 6. In: Richardson MJ, Riley MA, Shockley K (eds) Progress in motor control. Springer, New York
Nolte J, Sundsten JW (2002) The human brain: an introduction to its functional anatomy. Mosby, St. Louis
Nyce DS (2004) Linear position sensors: theory and application. Wiley, Hoboken
Opensim. http://opensim.stanford.edu
Paine NA (2014) High performance series elastic actuation. Ph.D. dissertation, University of Texas at Austin, Austin
Panasonic. http://na.industrial.panasonic.com/sites/default/pidsa/files/downloads/files/panasonic_overview_information_on_li-ion_batteries.pdf
Petak JL (2014) Performance testing of a musculoskeletal model controller for a robotic prosthesis. Masters of Science thesis, Northern Arizona University, Department of Mechanical Engineering, Flagstaff
Petak J, Heckathorn N, LeMoyne R, Dyer J, Yeo SH, Pai D, Tester J, Nishikawa K (2013a) Winding filament muscle model for musculo-skeltal simulations. Proceedings of 37th annual meeting of the American Society of Biomechanics, Omaha, pp 1–2
Petak J, Heckathorne N, LeMoyne R, Dyer J, Yeo SH, Pai D, Tester J, Nishikawa K (2013b) A new muscle model for neuro-musculo-skeletal simulations. Proceedings of 8th annual dynamic walking conference, Pittsburgh, p 1
Pratt GA, Williamson MM (1995) Series elastic actuators. Proceedings of IEEE international conference on intelligent robots and systems 95. 'Human Robot Interaction and Cooperative Robots', Pittsburgh, pp 399–406
Robinson DW (2000) Design and analysis of series elasticity in closed-loop actuator force control. Ph.D. dissertation, MIT, Department of Mechanical Engineering, Cambridge
Seeley RR, Stephens TD, Tate P (2003) Anatomy & physiology. McGraw-Hill, New York
Stephan AM, Nahm KS (2006) Review on composite polymer electrolytes for lithium batteries. Polymer 47:5952–5964
Sutton GP (1992) Rocket propulsion elements: an introduction to the engineering of rockets. Wiley-Interscience, New York
Tester J, Yeo SH, Pai D, Nishikawa K (2012) A new muscle model with implications for actuation and control. Proceedings of 7th annual dynamic walking conference, Pensacola Beach, pp 1–3
Thelen DG (2003) Adjustment of muscle mechanics model parameters to simulate dynamic contractions in older adults. J Biomech Eng 125:70–77

Wang K, McClure J, Tu A (1979) Titin: major myofibrillar components of striated muscle. Proc Natl Acad Sci U S A 76:3698–3702

Watson C, Kirkcaldie M, Paxinos G (2010) The brain: an introduction to functional neuroanatomy. Academic Press, New York

Yeo SH (2012) Computational modeling of neuromusculoskeletal systems: from filaments to behavior. Ph.D. dissertation, University of British Columbia (Vancouver), Department of Computer Science, Vancouver

Zajac FE (1989) Muscle and tendon: properties, models, scaling, and application to biomechanics and motor control. Crit Rev Biomed Eng 17:359–411

Zlatnik D, Steiner B, Schweitzer G (2002) Finite-state control of a trans-femoral (TF) prosthesis. IEEE Trans Control Syst Technol 10:408–420

Chapter 8
Transtibial Powered Prostheses: Single and Dual Actuator Configurations

Abstract The actuator derived powered prosthesis configuration enables a diversity of contextually specified applications. Current configurations incorporate single and dual actuator strategies. These types of powered prostheses satisfy mission specific objectives. Single actuator powered prosthetic designs generally enable powered plantar flexion and actuator established control of the prosthetic ankle-foot complex. Another unique single actuator powered prosthesis emphasizes dorsiflexion control primarily enabling toe clearance during swing phase. With trend toward miniaturization dual actuator configuration powered prostheses are now feasible. These powered prostheses provide more biomimetic representation as the ankle-foot complex is inherently segmented. Dual actuator powered prostheses have been demonstrated to provide further advances respective of lifestyle activity opportunities.

Keywords Series elastic actuator • Powered plantar flexion • Single actuator configuration • Dual actuator configuration • Segmented ankle-foot complex

8.1 Introduction

As covered in the previous Chap. 2: 'Ankle-foot complex and the fundamental aspects of gait', the intact ankle-foot complex imparts substantial majority of the mechanical energy to the gait cycle during the terminal phase of stance. Chapters 5: 'Passive transtibial prosthesis and associated prosthetic components' and 6: 'Energy Storage and Return (ESAR) prosthesis' demonstrate previous decades of steady transition from the conventional post World War 2 Solid Ankle Cushioned Heel (SACH) to prostheses, such as the Seattle Foot and Flex-Foot, that store and return a portion of energy throughout the span of the stance phase have been realized. Prosthetic technology has progressively advanced with the discovery of the significance of powered plantar flexion for gait during the 1980s by Winter (Winter 1983; Winter and Sienko 1988; LeMoyne 2015).

The currently powered prosthesis designs address two types of configurations depending on the objectives of the research and development team. These two types of configurations addressed involve single actuator and dual actuator powered

R. LeMoyne, *Advances for Prosthetic Technology*,
DOI 10.1007/978-4-431-55816-3_8

prostheses. Both of these configurations enable unique opportunities for the user of the powered prosthesis.

8.2 Single Actuator Configuration of Transtibial Powered Prosthesis

8.2.1 Proprio Foot

Another actuator facilitated type of transtibial prosthesis is the Proprio Foot developed by Ossur. The design of the Proprio Foot is envisioned to enhance dorsiflexion during the swing phase of gait cycle. The proper level of dorsiflexion during swing phase reduces the probability stumbling, which cannot be modulated for a fixed position passive prosthesis. Correct dorsiflexion about the ankle joint also facilitates heel strike during the initiation of stance phase. A linear actuator provides power about the ankle joint for dorsiflexion (Fradet et al. 2010; Darter and Wilken 2014; Ossur).

The appropriate level of dorsiflexion is determined through a microprocessor that operates an artificial intelligence platform. An angle sensor and accelerometers provide the afferent acuity to the artificial intelligence system for establishing the desired dorsiflexion about the prosthetic ankle joint. This sensory feedback is achieved through a high sampling rate (Fradet et al. 2010; Darter and Wilken 2014; Ossur).

Preliminary testing and evaluation of the Ossur Proprio Foot has been demonstrated through multiple gait analysis systems. Gait kinematics and kinetics have been applied through the use of motion capture devices and force plates. Initial experimentation has demonstrated the capacity of the Ossur Proprio Foot to adapt to ramp ascent scenarios, underscores the prosthesis' ability to acclimate to non-level gait conditions (Fradet et al. 2010). Other gait analysis has been applied to assessing improvements regarding metabolic expenditure, for which partial success was revealed in the context of level, inclined, and declined walking environments (Darter and Wilken 2014).

However, the Ossur Proprio Foot is designed to provide active dorsiflexion not any power about the plantar flexion aspect of stance. During stance this prosthesis functions in a manner comparable to passive elastic prosthesis with the prosthetic ankle joint in a fixed position (Au et al. 2007a, b; Au 2007; Gates et al. 2013). The implication is that no mechanical actuated work is contributed to the gait cycle during stance phase (LeMoyne 2015).

8.2.2 AMP-Foot 2.0

An alternative configuration for a single actuator powered prosthesis is to store energy with the progressive function of a lower power actuator with higher power release at the proper subphase of stance. This concept entails a low power actuator that stores energy in the form of a spring assembly, and then facilitates sudden release of the energy in a shorter time frame, which permits a higher power for the shorter time frame. Cherrelle et al. have developed such a powered prosthesis using a single low power actuator know as the AMP-Foot 2.0 (Cherelle et al. 2012).

The primary design of objective of the AMP-Foot 2.0 is to store energy through a dual spring system, with a low power actuator that contributes additional energy to the terminal phase of the gait cycle. One spring is termed the plantar flexion spring. This spring connects to an aspect of the prosthetic foot to a lever arm through a cable that passes through a pulley mounted to the foot. The plantar flexion spring stores energy during the controlled dorsiflexion aspect of stance (Cherelle et al. 2012).

The other spring is referred to as the push off spring, and energy is cumulatively stored through a low power actuator. With a locking system the push off spring is released in the terminal aspect of stance before heel off is achieved. The design incorporates two lever arms that interact with the spring. The advantage of this configuration is that the power requirements of the actuator can be reduced, since the energy release duration through the push off spring is shorter than the energy storage through the actuator (Cherelle et al. 2012).

The control architecture incorporates five states to encompass the gait cycle: heel strike to foot flat, foot flat to heel off, heel off, heel off to toe off, and swing phase. From heel strike to foot flat the plantar flexion spring extends, which provides a semblance of controlled plantar flexion with the torque produced. During this phase the low power actuator of the push off spring stores energy with the spring assembly. However, as the spring is in a locked status, no torque is imparted about the prosthetic ankle joint (Cherelle et al. 2012).

The next phase is from foot flat to heel off. The mechanical arrangement of the plantar flexion spring enables the AMP-Foot 2.0 to modulate stiffness, which resembles of the ankle-foot complex. During this phase the low power actuator is still storing potential energy in the push off spring (Cherelle et al. 2012).

At heel off the stored energy of the push off spring is provided to the terminal aspect of stance phase by releasing the locking mechanism. Both springs release their stored energy, which provide energy to the gait cycle. The sudden increase in torque about the ankle joint is accompanied with a decrease in stiffness. From heel off to toe off the ankle achieves an equilibrium position (Cherelle et al. 2012).

The final is swing phase. This phase involves the AMP-Foot 2.0 being reset to its initial status. The actuator proceeds in an opposite direction to the initial position. Return springs restore the ankle angular position to the original state. The locking mechanism is closed for the next heel strike (Cherelle et al. 2012).

The AMP-Foot 2.0 was envisioned for a person with a mass of 75 kg. The low power actuator requirements were satisfied with a Maxon RE 30 Brush DC motor rated at 60 W. The plantar flexion spring employed 29 belleville springs positioned in series. The push off spring consisted of two tension springs (Cherelle et al. 2012).

A unique feature of the AMP-Foot 2.0 is the locking mechanism. There are four requirements that the locking mechanism is intended to satisfy:

- Withstand high loads
- Compact and lightweight
- Capable of locking at a prescribed angle
- Unlock at maximum load environment (Cherelle et al. 2012)

A four bar linkage mechanism was selected with a solenoid for modulation. This mechanism has been successfully demonstrated (van Oort et al. 2011; Cherelle et al. 2012).

Multiple sensors ascertained gait status, and telemetry was wirelessly transmitted. Both spring assemblies incorporated strain gauges. The spatial position of the lever arms was determined through two absolute magnetic encoders. Two force sensing resistors mounted about the toes and heel aspect of the foot assembly determined the relationship with ground contact, such as heel strike (initial contact), foot flat, heel off, and toe off. The force sensing resistors provide control acuity respective of the status of the locking mechanism and low power actuator (Cherelle et al. 2012).

Future evolutions of the AMP-Foot 2.0 envision advances regarding the control system. Modifications to the activity of the low power actuator are envisioned to be beneficial. Reducing the force necessary to disengage the four bar mechanism would be advantageous to the overall design (Cherelle et al. 2012).

Preliminary test and evaluation of the AMP-Foot 2.0 has revealed biomimetic qualities that are essential aspects of human gait. The AMP-Foot 2.0 demonstrates a similar torque versus angle profile relative to the ankle-foot complex during gait cycle. In particular, the stance phase of the ankle-foot complex is encompassed in the AMP-Foot 2.0 torque versus angle profile (Cherelle et al. 2012).

Another significant capability of the AMP-Foot 2.0 exhibited by preliminary testing and evaluation is the ankle power as a function of stride time. The intact ankle-foot complex displays considerable power output during the terminal phase of stance. The low power actuator progressively stores energy, but the actuator functions at a lower power setting notably less than the peak power output of the ankle-foot complex. As the stored energy in the push off spring is released the AMP-Foot 2.0 produces considerable power during the terminal phase of stance, which even transcends the power output of the representative ankle-foot complex (Cherelle et al. 2012).

In summary this type of powered prosthesis for people with transtibial amputation demonstrates the feasibility of low power actuators for generating representative ankle power during stance. The AMP-Foot 2.0 incorporates a two spring system. One spring stores energy with the loading of the ankle during stance, and the other spring is progressively stored with potential energy through the low power actuator. The spring with the potential energy as a result of the actuator is released at the appropriate time through a locking mechanism (Cherelle et al. 2012).

8.2.3 *Kanazawa Institute of Technology Powered Prosthesis*

Suzuki et al. developed a powered prosthesis for people with transtibial amputation. The design features an internal control model for regulating the gait cycle. The pattern for the pending gait cycle is established as a function of the previous gait sequence. A unique characteristic of this concept is the control system does not require force sensors or pressure sensors (Suzuki et al. 2011).

Along with the internal control model the device developed by Suzuki et al. is comprised of standard components for a powered prosthesis. Respective of actuator subsystems the powered prosthesis consists of a DC motor and motor driver, which is powered by a localized battery. Sensing acuity is enabled through a rotary encoder. The control system is evaluated through a microcomputer with control about the ankle joint facilitated through a tendon-drive mechanism. The aggregate mass of the powered prosthesis inclusive of the battery is approximately 3.8 kg (Suzuki et al. 2011).

The control architecture is established through the standard gait cycle, which is comprised of transition from stance to swing. In terms of the stance phase, there are three defined subphases defined as mode 1 to mode 3, which have previously been established by Au et al. during 2008:

- Mode 1 (controlled plantar flexion): The research team of Suzuki interprets mode 1 as spanning from heel strike to foot flat.
- Mode 2 (controlled dorsiflexion): For mode 2 Suzuki et al. infer this subphase commences at foot flat and continues to maximal dorsiflexion. This aspect of stance encompasses the storage of energy, which augments mode 3.
- Mode 3 (powered plantarflexion): Mode 3 transitions from the end of maximal dorsiflexion to toe off. This subphase is comprised of the release of stored elastic energy from mode 2 and powered plantar flexion (Au et al. 2008; Suzuki et al. 2011).

The interpretations of mode 1 through mode 3 are envisioned as sufficient to emulate stance phase with the internal control model developed by Suzuki et al. (Au et al. 2008; Suzuki et al. 2011).

The efficacy of the powered prosthesis and its supporting internal control model has been experimentally corroborated both with visual interpretation and sensor data from the rotary encoder positioned at the ankle joint. In particular the ankle mounted rotary encoder enables the activation of powered plantar flexion upon a threshold of 8° (positive) in dorsiflexion. This phase is terminated once the plantar flexion orientation attains a threshold between 15° and 18° (negative). The experimental findings of Suzuki et al. advocate the sufficiency of their powered prosthesis utilizing and internal control model scheme for imparting adequate mechanical energy to the gait cycle during the terminal phase of stance (Suzuki et al. 2011).

8.3 Dual Actuator Configurations of Transtibial Powered Prostheses

As actuators are progressively miniaturized, the capacity to encapsulate more than one actuator within the packaging constraints of the transtibial prosthesis is feasible. For example, an actuator can be positioned to emulate the large toe during terminal stance phase, benefiting the user's energy efficiency and gait symmetry (Zhu et al. 2010). Parallel aligned actuators placed in the tibial aspect of the powered prosthesis are envisioned to provide another powered degree of freedom, such as ankle inversion and eversion (Bellman et al. 2008). Dual configuration actuators for powered transtibial prosthetic systems have even been demonstrated from proof of concept for restoration of running capability. Such configurations are envisioned for the exceptional goal of facilitating soldiers with unilateral amputation to return to activity duty service for their country (Hitt et al. 2010).

These dual actuator prostheses address additional aspects of the gait cycle beyond the single actuator design. With the shift in objective, they also incorporate unique control architecture. Their contribution of the domain of highly advanced multi-actuator powered prosthesis warrants their representation.

8.3.1 PANTOE

From the perspective of the SACH, energy storage and return, and even the BiOM powered prosthesis; the foot aspect of a prosthetic system is approximated as a solid and singular structure with varying degrees of rigidity (Wilson 1963; Burgess et al. 1985; BiOM). However as clearly defined in Chap. 2: 'Ankle-foot complex and the fundamental aspects of gait', the foot is readily capable of ambulation with associated musculature. A future prosthetic designer can readily infer that improving biomimetic features specific to the prosthetic foot would likely advance a user's gait experience.

Zhu et al. proposes a powered prosthesis for people with transtibial amputation called PANTOE. The acronym PANTOE symbolizes a powered prosthesis with Powered Ankle and Toe Joints. In addition to mechanical actuation for powered plantar flexion amalgamates another actuator for the toe joint through a segmented foot (Zhu et al. 2010). Research has ascertained the benefit of a segmented foot configuration as the human foot is not representational of a singular rigid body. A segmented foot consisting of a toe joint provides utility to the gait cycle with regards to joint angle range of motion, angular velocity, and joint energy output

(Okita et al. 2009). The PANTOE is envisioned to further advance gait fidelity for transtibial amputees (Zhu et al. 2010).

The PANTOE powered prosthesis incorporates the contribution of the forefoot during stance phase. This unique dual actuator configuration requires the further refinement of the gait cycle during the stance phase, which encompasses 60 % of the entire gait cycle. Zhu et al. characterizes stance into four subphases:

- Heel strike to foot flat; The ankle-foot complex withstands impact and stores energy respective of the plantar flexor muscles.
- Foot flat to midstance; In this subphase the subsequently stored energy is released with center of gravity transition from support leg to foreleg.
- Midstance to heel off; During midstance the ankle-foot complex stores energy about the dorsiflexion musculature, until maximal ankle dorsiflexion is attained at the heel off threshold.
- Heel off to toe off; The ankle releases stored energy from the prior subphase. The ankle-foot complex imparts positive work to the gait cycle, such as through plantar flexor musculature. However, in the context of a segmented foot model, the forefoot also contributes to the energy enhancement to gait (Zhu et al. 2010).

The forefoot regulates energy contribution to the gait cycle in a fashion similar to the ankle and its musculature. During the heel off to toe off stance subphase, the forefoot stores energy while the joint is progressively rotated. At the terminal aspect of this subphase the stored energy is released with some supplemental positive work facilitating the gait cycle (Zhu et al. 2010).

With these features of gait established Zhu et al. established four primary design objectives:

- Incorporate a segmented powered prosthesis with joints about the ankle and forefoot to emulate human gait.
- Enable both joints to release stored energy while also imparting positive work to gait.
- Design the powered prosthesis, such that the device is analogous to the geometric and mass characteristics of the amputated limb.
- Establish maximal joint angle thresholds for the powered prosthesis:
  - 22° for the plantar flexion
  - 12° for dorsiflexion
  - 90° about the toe joint (Zhu et al. 2010)

In order to satisfy these design objectives and realistically emulate the human ankle-foot complex the research team of Zhu et al. needed to address design challenges of a considerable nature. Particular issues for biomimetic powered ankle-foot prosthesis pertain to the selection of the actuators and power source. The actuators constitute the prime movers of the powered prosthesis, such as for powered plantar flexion, and in the case of this particular prosthesis mechanical energy about the toe joint. The down selection for the actuator subsystem were primarily influenced in consideration of the following observations:

- Satisfy realistic volume and mass constraints for a lower limb transtibial amputation prosthesis
- Sufficient shock tolerance for imitating the behavior the ankle-foot complex (Zhu et al. 2010)

Synergistic to the proper selection of the actuators is the acquisition the power source. Essentially the actuators enable mechanical energy about the stance phase of gait; however, the actuators require a preliminary electrical power source, such as a battery. Likewise the power source selection should satisfy particular criteria:

- Sufficient energy to enable the user to engage in activities, such as effectively unrestricted walking distance for the scope of a day.
- In light of providing sufficient energy the mass properties should be realistic for a user with transtibial amputation (Zhu et al. 2010).

Based on these design constraints the research team of Zhu et al. selected two series elastic actuators powered by a lithium battery. Both series elastic actuators incorporated a DC motor attached to a transmission and spring. The selection of the series elastic actuators for enabling power about the ankle and toe joint was due to several factors:

- Back-drive capability and lower output impedance
- Enhanced shock tolerance because of the alignment of the spring in series with the transmission and load
- Improved energy efficiency with the kinetic and potential energy properties of the spring constituting an elastic element
- Advanced force control and stability
- Reduction in force requirements (Zhu et al. 2010)

The advantages of the lithium battery are its low cost, energy density, and rechargeable capability (Zhu et al. 2010).

The frame of the PANTOE1 prototype consisted of aluminum alloy, for the intent of minimizing aggregate mass. Overall the PANTOE1 had a mass of 1.47 kg. This mass was exclusive of the molded socket and rechargeable lithium battery (Zhu et al. 2010).

The power requirements for the ankle joint series elastic actuator are greater than for the toe joint series elastic actuator. The series elastic actuator for representing actuation about the ankle joint consisted of a power of 83 W for a DC motor accompanied with three parallel spring with a stiffness of 500 N/cm. As the toe joint requires reduced power about the joint a smaller actuator is warranted. The power for the toe joint actuator is 30 W for a DC motor comprised with four drawsprings in parallel orientation representing a stiffness of 200 N/cm. In particular to the toe joint actuator assembly, counterclockwise rotation is passive and clockwise rotation actively engages the actuator (Zhu et al. 2010).

Feedback is enabled through a sequence of sensors. These sensors provide significant information for the control system. Walking status of the subject is acquired, and the control system can be further optimized (Zhu et al. 2010).

A force sensor measures force at the interface of the subject and the PANTOE1 powered prosthesis. Angular orientation about the ankle joint is acquired through an angular encoder. At the toe segment a linear potentiometer is applied to obtain rotation angle and also the force applied against the springs in the toe series elastic actuator. Two contact sensors are positioned at both aspects of the segmented foot, the heel and toe assemblies (Zhu et al. 2010).

The preliminary control architecture for PANTOE1 involved controlling output torque as a function of rotational orientation of the ankle joint and its respective motor assembly. During the stance phase of gait the segmented joints of the powered prosthesis torque and position are controlled by a mutual relationship. However for swing phase the control system functions based on position (Zhu et al. 2010).

PANTOE1 incorporates three operational models to accommodate the user. Model 1 accounts for the scenario of the battery running out of power. During model 1 the PANTOE1 operates as a passive prosthesis as both motors are not operational. Model 2 is envisioned for lower power scenarios. For model 2 the series elastic actuator about the toe joint is not functioning, and the ankle joint actuator only modulates the angular position during swing phase. However, the series springs in both actuators are capable of storing and releasing energy during gait (Zhu et al. 2010).

Model 3 involves the synchronous use of both the series elastic actuator positioned at the ankle joint and toe joint. Upon preliminary heel strike the springs located in the series elastic actuator for the ankle stores energy until foot flat while also ameliorating shock from the prosthesis making contact with the ground. From foot flat to midstance stored energy is released. Between midstance to heel off the same spring component stores energy through extension. As the prosthesis proceeds from heel off to toe off, the stored energy of the corresponding spring is released while the series elastic actuator imparts energy respective of the ankle joint to the stance phase of gait. Positive energy is released to the stance phase of gait through the synergistic release of elastic energy and motor derived energy through the series elastic actuator at the toe joint. When swing phase is reached both series elastic actuators regulate angular orientation for the ankle joint and toe joint. In summary model 3 is envisioned to be the most interactive implementation between the user and the PANTOE1 powered prosthesis (Zhu et al. 2010).

Preliminary experimentation to establish the efficacy of the PANTOE1 concept was conducted by simulated walking. As illustrated in the research manuscript, an experimenter held the socket adaptor by hand and guided the PANTOE1 throughout the gait cycle from stance to swing. Based on visual contrast the PANTOE1 successfully emulated the human gait cycle. Future test and evaluation forecasts human usage of the PANTOE1 and further advances of the control system (Zhu et al. 2010).

8.3.2 Evolution of PANTOE

By 2014 Zhu et al. further evolved the PANTOE concept. The 2014 version of the PANTOE likewise identified five subphases of the stance phase for the human gait cycle: heel strike, foot flat, midstance, heel off, and toe off. The algorithm governing the PANTOE for this version was linearized trajectory control. Further refinement of both the ankle and toe torque and angle relationship is warranted (Zhu et al. 2014).

There are four segments that characterize the torque and angle relationship of the ankle. Between heel strike to foot flat the stiffness of the ankle joint decreases to absorb impact shock from contact. From foot flat to ankle maximum dorsiflexion ankle stiffness increases more rapidly with increasing angle, which represents energy storage for pending push off. As the ankle-foot complex proceeds to toe off angle stiffness decreases while ankle angle decreases, implicating the release of energy. The final phase from toe off to the next heel strike signifies the swing phase of gait. The ankle stiffness is essentially zero; however, the ankle angular orientation resets to a ready position for pending heel strike (Zhu et al. 2014).

The ankle joint torque and angle relationship's graphical representation proceeds in a counterclockwise manner. The counterclockwise nature of the curve constitutes the summation of positive work by the ankle joint. The positive work can be calculated according to the enclosed area of the torque and angle relationship (Zhu et al. 2014).

The toe joint torque to angle relationship is also comprised of four inherent aspects. During the first aspect the ankle-foot complex transitions from heel strike to foot flat to heel off, and the toe joint angle sustains effectively a zero orientation while the torque rapidly increases. From heel off to toe joint maximal dorsiflexion the toe angle increases and the torque increases at an attenuating rate. As the toe joint transitions to toe off torque is released as both toe angle and toe torque decrease. During the swing cycle transition from toe off to pending heel strike the toe stiffness and joint orientation reset to effectively zero (Zhu et al. 2014).

The mechanical design of the 2014 version of the PANTOE resembles the 2010 prototype. Both the ankle joint and toe joint were equipped with series elastic actuators (Zhu et al. 2010, 2014). In order to accommodate a 70 kg person for the current PANTOE incorporates a higher spring stiffness of 1800 N/cm for the ankle series elastic actuator. The PANTOE also incorporates a tethered battery configuration. The user wears a waist-mounted belt attached to a rechargeable lithium battery, which connects to the PANTOE through a tethered cable. A linearized trajectory control strategy is incorporated due to its robust nature (Zhu et al. 2014).

Zhu et al. identified two primary design drivers for selecting linearized trajectory control. The simplicity of this control strategy facilitates a reduced response time. Any delay in processing time during a subject's walking could produce hazards that increase the likelihood of a fall. Also the transition from state to state is achieved by straight-line segments, which can be easily adjusted by modifying their associated slopes. This perspective is envisioned to facilitate the adaptation of control parameters for an assortment of walking speeds (Zhu et al. 2014).

Linearized trajectory control models the ankle joint through six straight-line segments. The control strategy features two straight-lines to transition from toe off to heel strike and heel strike to foot flat. Due to the curvature between the transitions from foot flat to ankle maximum dorsiflexion and ankle maximum dorsiflexion to toe off, two straight lines are incorporated to approximate both transitions with an intermediary point for each transition (Zhu et al. 2014).

The sensor platform greatly facilitates the implementation of the control strategy. The PANTOE incorporated to conventional contact switches at the heel and forefoot. These sensors identified heel strike, foot flat, heel off, and toe off. Two angle sensors (circular-shaped potentiometers) were applied to acquire spatial orientation for the joint angle and toe angle (Zhu et al. 2014).

8.3.3 Human Testing of PANTOE

Human testing of the PANTOE powered prosthesis was commenced with regards to one subject with transtibial amputation. The experiment contrasted a conventional passive prosthesis (1S90, Ottobock) relative to the PANTOE powered prosthesis. The subject was tasked to walk at a speed of 1.25 m/s, which was interpreted as within a comfortable threshold. A total of ten gait cycles were collected for each prosthetic scenario (Zhu et al. 2014).

The gait analysis equipment was selected to measure two gait parameters: joint angle and ground reaction force. These objectives were achieved through the use of a Footscan force plate by RSscan Inc. and a Codamotion 3D motion analysis system by Charnwood Dynamics Ltd. Presented results were based on the averaging of all ten gait trials and contrasted to the intact lower limb (Zhu et al. 2014).

With regards to the intact lower limb contrasted to the limb with the passive prosthesis, the knee joint angle orientations display graphically comparable trends about the entire gait cycle. However the ankle angle and toe angle for both the intact and passive prosthesis limb is effectively asymmetric. Also the toe angle maximal dorsiflexion is considerably reduced for the passive prosthesis relative to the intact limb (Zhu et al. 2014).

Asymmetry is notably pronounced for the ground reaction force during stance phase. The passive prosthesis initiates stance with a load on the order of roughly three times exceeding the intact limb. The passive prosthesis also displays diminished reaction force about the terminal aspect of stance compared to the intact limb (Zhu et al. 2014). These gait biomechanical observations are indicative of progressive and chronically degenerative morbidities (LeMoyne 2015).

The PANTOE enables considerable restoration to the subject's gait kinematics and kinetics. All three joint angles about the knee, ankle, and toe demonstrate relatively symmetric kinematic profiles relative to the intact limb. The most significant improvement is with regards to the ground reaction force profile for both the residual leg with the PANTOE prosthesis and the intact leg (Zhu et al. 2014).

The ground reaction force signal of both the leg with PANTOE prosthesis and intact leg are relatively symmetrical. The initial stance phase for the PANTOE is more appropriately reduced compared to the passive prosthesis and scalable to the intact limb. Also the push off aspect of terminal gait is highly similar while demonstrating an appropriate magnitude (Zhu et al. 2014). The successful observations of preliminary test and evaluation reveal the biomimetic and sustainable features of the PANTOE.

In addition to the success from a biomechanical perspective of gait, the subject commented the perception of feeling more comfortable and agile while walking with PANTOE by contrast to the passive prosthesis. Future evolutions of PANTOE envision the implementation of more advanced control strategies. For example, the control parameters could be adapted to particular gait scenarios, such as through learning algorithms (Zhu et al. 2014).

8.3.4 Control Strategy for PANTOE

With the mechanical design of the PANTOE successfully demonstrated through the dual series elastic actuator implementation about the ankle joint and toe joint, evolutions emphasize the development of an advanced control strategy (Yuan et al. 2011). Finite state control strategies have been previously developed from ankle joint only series elastic actuator configurations (Au et al. 2007a, b, 2009, Au 2007). The research and development team evolving the PANTOE envisions the development of a finite state control strategy for a dual actuator powered ankle joint and toe joint. Future efforts plan to establish a control strategy that is provides stable interaction between subject, powered prosthesis, and environment; but also the capacity to mitigate abnormal gait disturbances (Yuan et al. 2011).

The control architecture is developed with the four subphase aspects of stance phase of gait that were previously established for the development of PANTOE:

1. Heel Strike to Foot Flat
2. Foot Flat to Midstance
3. Midstance to Heel Off
4. Heel Off to Toe Off (Yuan et al. 2011)

For this control architecture the most significant involvement of the toe joint is during the heel off to toe off subphase. In the preliminary aspect of this subphase the toe joint undergoes dorsiflexion, as energy is stored. Upon the terminal part of transition to toe off, the toe joint releases stored energy and imparts positive work to the gait cycle (Yuan et al. 2011).

In order to implement the proposed control architecture, the following sensors are included to provide feedback:

- Two contact switches are positioned beneath the heel and toe, respectively. The purpose of these sensors is to define foot position relative to the ground surface.
- Two force sensors that are also located beneath the heel and toe. Their objective is to derive pressure about the heel and toe.
- Two circular shaped potentiometers are located at the ankle joint and toe joint to determine angular orientation for both joints.
- A linear potentiometer is placed parallel to the ankle spring, in order to approximate ankle torque (Yuan et al. 2011).

A timer in the control chip measures time, and estimates time allocated to swing phase and stance phase of gait. The controller incorporates seven input/output ports. With these sensors ankle angle velocity is computed by the differential of angular orientation. An ankle joint series elastic actuator rated at 83 W and a toe joint series elastic actuator rated at 45 W facilitates this control architecture. The actuators incorporate DC motors by Faulhaber (Yuan et al. 2011).

The finite state control architecture is defined by seven discrete states that encompass the representation of stance and swing phase.

1. Controlled plantar flexion of ankle
2. Controlled dorsiflexion of ankle
3. Powered plantar flexion of ankle
4. Controlled dorsiflexion of toe
5. Powered plantar flexion of toe
6. Early swing
7. Late swing (Yuan et al. 2011)

The strategy for the finite state control of the PANTOE is derived from the successful process developed by Zlantik et al. (2002). Finite state control proceeds to another state upon satisfying prescribed transition thresholds. Transition from controlled plantar flexion of ankle (1) to controlled dorsiflexion of ankle (2) requires three requirements to be satisfied. Heel and toe are in ground contact ($\mathrm{H}=1, \mathrm{T}=1$). Heel-strike to toe-strike time interval is constrained by a defined time interval ($\Delta \mathrm{t} > \mathrm{t_p}$). Ankle joint angle is greater than zero ($\Theta_a > 0$) (Yuan et al. 2011).

At controlled dorsiflexion of ankle (2) there are three criteria to transition to powered plantar flexion of ankle (3). The heel must be off the ground ($\mathrm{H}=0$). The angular velocity about the ankle joint is less than zero ($\dot{\Theta}_a < 0$). Ankle torque must exceed a prescribed threshold ($T_a > \tau_{pp}$) (Yuan et al. 2011).

At state 3 powered plantar flexion of ankle the transition to controlled dorsiflexion of the toe (4) occurs by satisfying the threshold that toe angle exceeds a threshold of zero ($\Theta_t > 0$). For states 1, 2, 3, and 4 transition to a stop mode can be achieved through both heel and toe being off the ground ($\mathrm{H}=0$, $\mathrm{T}=0$) (Yuan et al. 2011).

Transition from state 4 controlled dorsiflexion of the toe to state 5 powered plantar flexion of the toe is achieved by two requirements. Toe angle must transcend a prescribed threshold ($\Theta_t > \Theta_p$). Toe pressure exceeds a predefined threshold ($F_T > F_{PT}$) (Yuan et al. 2011).

After the powered plantar flexion of toe (5), early swing (6) commences. There are two requirements regarding ground contact. Both the heel and toe must be off the ground (H = 0, T = 0). In the event that the PANTOE is in stop mode, and both heel and toe are contacting the ground (H = 1, T = 1), then the PANTOE transitions from stop mode to early swing at state 6 (Yuan et al. 2011).

Early swing (6) transitions to late swing (7) when the angle about the ankle equals zero ($\Theta_a = 0$). In order to transition back to state 1 controlled plantar flexion, there are four threshold criteria. Both angular orientation and angular velocity regarding the ankle must be less than zero ($\dot{\Theta}_a < 0$ and $\Theta_a < 0$). The heel must be in contact with the ground (H = 1), and heel pressure must exceed a prescribed threshold ($F_H > F_{PH}$) (Yuan et al. 2011).

This finite state architecture is envisioned not only to enable the fluid transition through gait subphases, but also mitigate the effect of abnormal gait situations. The toe pressure threshold ($F_T > F_{PT}$) is intended to facilitate the user while standing on the heel but not intending to walk forward. The interval between heel to toe strike ($\Delta t > t_p$) is designed to prevent initiation of forward motion when the subject strikes the PANTOE to the ground. In the event of a slip, the heel and toe off (H = 0 and T = 0) are designed to transition to stop state. Then upon standing with full foot contact (H = 1 and T = 1) PANTOE resets to early swing phase (6). Another utility of this finite state control is that based on stance time or swing time, the total time period of the gait cycle can be acquired. Therefore, the control architecture can adapt to variations in gait speed (Yuan et al. 2011).

The control strategy proceeds about the following sequence. The PANTOE resets to an equilibrium state once started. The equilibrium state initialized the toe angle and ankle angle to zero. Walking speed is initialized based on stance or swing time. Then the sensors are scanned to ascertain whether the transition threshold criteria are attained. In the event that the criteria are satisfied, a new state's transition occurs. Otherwise the sensors are again scanned. The new states sequence of commands is executed. The time interval between two adjacent states feeds back to the determination of speed initialization. This sequence continues until the end of operation (Yuan et al. 2011).

Simulated experimentation determined the efficacy of the PANTOE's finite state control strategy to identify and transition among the seven states of the PANTOE prescribed gait cycle. The researchers envision future test and evaluation by people with unilateral transtibial amputation to further establish the efficacy of the control architecture. Further advances are planned to develop finite control strategies that are also amendable for climbing and descending stairs (Yuan et al. 2011).

8.3.5 Spring Ankle with Regenerative Kinetics (SPARKy)

A research team led by Arizona State University has developed a powered prosthesis configuration termed Spring Ankle with Regenerative Kinetics (SPARKy).

The objective of the endeavor was to restore ankle-foot complex functionality in the context of gait to persons with amputation, and even enable soldiers with amputation to return to active duty service. The SPARKy powered prosthesis has been progressively evolved over multiple phases with the first evolution consisting of a singular actuator arrangement and the third evolution enabling a dual actuator configuration (Bellman et al. 2008; Holgate et al. 2008).

The primary components of the SPARKy powered prosthesis are the spring keel representing the foot, lever arm, pylon, and Robotic Tendon. The Robotic Tendon consists of a lightweight actuator. The actuator is comprised of primarily an efficient DC motor, helical springs, and a robust position controller (Holgate et al. 2008). This actuator design architecture is comparable to the series elastic actuator previously designed by MIT (Pratt and Williamson 1995).

During the stance phase of gait the Robotic Tendon is capable of storing energy during the preliminary aspect of stance. The stored potential energy of the spring facilitates the robotic tendon by mitigating the need for a traditional higher power motor. The spring releases its energy in synchronicity with the actuator for the peak power aspect of push off during stance. This approach considerably reduces power requirements for the motor (Hollander et al. 2005; Holgate et al. 2008).

Actuator requirements of the Robotic Tendon are further relieved with the addition of a parallel unidirectional spring. The parallel unidirectional spring provides utility to the SPARKy powered prosthesis during the phase of stance that involves dorsiflexion of the foot, and this spring is oriented in parallel to the Robotic Tendon. The role of the parallel unidirectional spring is to decrease actuator energy requirements, such as during slow and average (self-selected) walking speeds (Holgate et al. 2008). This design amendment has also been successfully implemented by researchers at MIT (Au et al. 2007a, b; Au 2007).

The SPARKy research and development process continued and produced three types of progressively improved powered prostheses. Following the development of the first SPARKy powered prosthesis a half year of subject test and evaluation ensued. Pending improvements based on the test and evaluation were applied. The mass was reduced from 2.7 kg for the original SPARKy to 2.0 kg for the SPARKy 2. Improvements emphasize the linear transmission such as incorporating a ball screw or roller screw and a more powerful and compact brushless motor that did not require a gearbox (Bellman et al. 2008).

The evolution of the SPARKy 3 is projected to enable the athletic capabilities intrinsic with the requirements for an active duty soldier and people who seek a considerable level of personal activity. Most powered prosthetic applications enable power about the sagittal plane, which is the predominant plane for general gait. However, facilitating powered actuation about the coronal plane would empower the user with more complex human movements, such as dorso-ventral, elevational, and transverse body movements. The SPARKy 3 design is capable of two degrees of freedom through the addition of two joints and two actuators (Bellman et al. 2008).

The primary design objective of the SPARKy 3 was to develop a powered prosthesis with considerable dynamic ability, without compromising the performance of previous evolutions or prohibitive increase in mass and volume. The foot aspect of the powered prosthesis was a LP Vari-Flex foot produced by Ossur, which enables a low clearance keel that contains two bolts that are amenable for mounting helical springs of the SPARKy (Bellman et al. 2008).

These helical springs are either extended or compressed through the two motors. Two Maxon EC Powermax 30 motor was selected for powering the prosthesis. Each motor has a continuous output power of 200 W, and tandem operation may attain a threshold of 1000 W. Synergy with the Robotic Tendon configuration is envisioned to provide peak power of 1500 W feasible and also 200 Nm of torque viable. These two parameters are inherent for jogging and sprint initiation, respectively. In principle the springs and motors are designed to facilitate the release of power during the terminal aspect of stance phase (Bellman et al. 2008).

The SPARKy 3 is capable of providing rotation about the sagittal and coronal plane. The two degrees of freedom configuration is permitted through two rotational axes. The primary axis representative of the center of rotation for the ankle-foot complex is the sagittal plane that encompasses plantar flexion and dorsiflexion. The secondary axis provides inversion and eversion through an orthogonal U-joint. The linear displacement of the actuators was conveyed to the helical springs mounted on the foot using L-shaped arms that were denoted "L-arms" (Bellman et al. 2008).

The axis of motion of the SPARKy 3 powered prosthesis is determined by the functionality of the actuators. Rotation about the primary axis occurs with both actuators providing synchronized power. Inversion or eversion about the secondary axis can occur during a scenario that involves the two actuators providing power in disparate directions. The SPARKy 3 has an overall system mass of 2.1 kg (Bellman et al. 2008).

8.3.6 Bionic Prosthesis for Military Amputees

With the rapid procession of technology advances and evolution the scope of prosthetic systems have transcended a major threshold with the bionic prosthesis for military amputees. A bold precedent is established with its implied design objectives. The bionic prosthesis for military amputees is envisioned to facilitate soldiers with amputations to be able to return to active service. Respective of the United States of America, the Army Physical Fitness Test constitutes an imperative aspect for return to active service. An aspect of the Army Physical Fitness Test includes a level ground condition 2 mile run that satisfies a timed threshold (Hitt et al. 2010).

The objective to develop a bionic prosthesis for military amputees entails a multidisciplinary research team. The research team comprises faculty, staff, and cadets of the United States Military Academy of West Point, New York. Other research team member are inclusive of clinicians from Walter Reed Medical Center and private industry contribution from SpringActive Inc. This team has successfully demonstrated from a preliminary perspective a dual actuator architecture that is highly promising for satisfying the design objectives (Hitt et al. 2010).

The thresholds for a powered prosthetic design that satisfies military demands for active duty certainly exceeds the perceptible thresholds for a satisfactory design for any civilian active lifestyle. Intuitively the powered prosthesis should be advantageous to the user from a kinematic perspective and metabolically efficient. The application would need to be adaptable to a considerable array of environments and feasible for an assortment of terrain and weather scenarios. In the event that a passive prosthesis is sufficient, active components, such as the computer for the control system and actuator motor, should be removable. The prosthetic design should operate on a single battery charge per day and also integrate with the soldier's equipment package. The overall system architecture should be amenable to airborne and waterborne scenarios (Hitt et al. 2010).

The foundation to the preliminary test and evaluation of the bionic prosthetic for military amputees is derived from the SPARKy powered prosthesis for walking, which was developed by Hitt et al. The SPARKy powered prosthesis for walking was evolved to a powered prosthesis capable of sustained running. Primary revisions entailed modification to structural elements and an actuator assembly that satisfied power requirements for running (Hitt et al. 2010).

Finite element analysis revealed three aspects of the powered prosthesis that required revision. These three aspects were at interface settings, such as the robotic muscle tendon, tibia-ankle, and tendon-ankle. A dual actuator architecture with each actuator interacting with a single spring ameliorated excessive stress about the interfaces (Hitt et al. 2010).

The actuator power requirement for running mandated a power constraint in the range of 300 to 400 W. This design condition could either be satisfied by a single more powerful actuator or two tandem operated and relatively less powerful actuators. The selection of a suitable actuator level is dependent on multiple design considerations. A single actuator can excessive moments about the interface, such as the muscle tendon component. A dual actuator can mitigate the risk of mechanical failure about the interface. However a dual actuator application requires synchronization that imparts additional requirements to the control system level. The research team selected the Maxon RE40 as the most preferable compromise in consideration of efficiency and motor control (Hitt et al. 2010).

The preliminary control system architecture utilizes MATLAB as its primary software language for controlling the dual actuators. The hardware was comprised of a PC104 microprocessor utilizing a Sensoray DAQ. The hardware interacts with the position controllers for both actuators. The architecture employed Ethernet connectivity to a local PC for downloading of the control software and acquisition of telemetry data (Hitt et al. 2010).

The control software was derived from an algorithm developed by Holgate et al. The benefit of this is control perspective is that there is no discrete transition from walking to running. Instead, the algorithm is effectively continuous, since state decision logic is not incorporated (Holgate et al. 2009; Hitt et al. 2010).

The control system was established using a two-dimensional representation. A functional relationship between motor position and gait cycle in terms of position and stride length was developed. This two-dimensional functional relationship was applied to the control system memory, which constituted a lookup table for referencing motor position based on tibia spatial position (Hitt et al. 2010).

Preliminary testing and evaluation involved a United States Army Special Operations noncommissioned officer. The subject has a mass of 80 kg and a unilateral transtibial amputation. A sustained 8 mile per hour moderate run was achieved on a treadmill. Based on observations of the experimental apparatus, a support harness was incorporated during the run for safety purposes. Anecdotally the subject abruptly stopped after the run by jumping off the treadmill, underscoring the robustness of the dual actuator prosthesis (Hitt et al. 2010).

Future evolutions of the powered prosthetic design are envisioned. Weight reduction through increasing battery energy density and advanced manufacturing processes are projected. A future design objective would be to decrease the power needed to transcend inertia of structural components and the actuator. A redesign is foreseen to employ a roller screw configuration as opposed to a lead screw. Another future objective would be to increase the actuator power capability (Hitt et al. 2010).

8.3.7 Multi-actuator Configuration Enabling Agonist/ Antagonist Powered Prosthesis Strategy

Preliminary proof of concept has been commenced by Versluys et al. in the context of a multiple actuator design for a powered prosthesis. This endeavor permits a agonist/antagonist arrangement for emulating the ankle-foot complex with respect to both the plantar flexors and dorsiflexors. Rather than utilizing a battery powered system for electro-mechanical actuators, the transtibial prosthetic design by Versluys et al. is pneumatically actuated with a compressed air source (Versluys et al. 2009).

Although the pleated pneumatic artificial muscles require a pressure source, which implies a tethering source, the objective of providing representative torque during the gait cycle in the range of 200 Nm is viable. In order to provide this torque requirement, a pressure source on the scale of 3×10^5 Pascal is required. This pressure rating is on the order of the inflation pressure of a standard bicycle tire. Pleated pneumatic artificial muscle actuators are intrinsically compliant, considerably lightweight, and able to produce significant force. With these attractive features of the pleated pneumatic artificial muscle Versluys et al. believe that their pneumatically powered prosthesis can improve walking ability for people with transtibial amputation (Versluys et al. 2009).

The advantageous design attributes of the pleated pneumatic artificial muscle enables a multi-actuator configuration that is more demonstrative of the ankle-foot complex muscular morphology. The actuator level configuration incorporates three pleated pneumatic artificial muscle actuators. Two pneumatic actuators are positioned posteriorly to provide plantar flexion, and the third actuator is located at the anterior section of the powered prosthesis to produce dorsiflexion. The superior aspect of the pneumatic actuators is connected to the prosthetic socket, and the inferior aspect is attached to an Axtion foot developed by Otto Bock HealthCare from Germany. By visual inspection of the pneumatic powered prosthesis mounted to a person with amputation, the device has a slightly larger in terms of volume, relative to the intact leg. However, the packaging volume of the pneumatic powered prosthesis does not appear to induce any negative impacts regarding functional ambulation (Versluys et al. 2009).

The sensor level is comprised of three types: an encoder, pressure sensors, and footswitches. The role of the encoder is to measure angular position about the prosthetic ankle joint. Three pressure sensors were applied to the three pneumatic actuators to evaluate pneumatic pressure during operation. Three footswitches were located in at the prosthetic foot to determine gait status during stance phases. The first footswitch was mounted at the heel to determined initial contact of the foot. The second footswitch was placed near the forefoot to acquire the instance of toe-off. A third footswitch was situated between the first two footswitches for ascertaining dorsiflexion during midstance (Versluys et al. 2009).

As the objective of the research by Versluys et al. was to demonstrate the capabilities of the pleated pneumatic artificial muscle in the context of a powered prosthesis, the control architecture was fundamental in nature. The torque produced was not regulated by a feedback system, instead the control of the actuators were based on feed forward principles. Prescribed torque output was established as a function of voltage signals for the servo valves that controlled the pressure to the pleated pneumatic artificial muscles. The proper voltage signal was applied to correspond with the walking requirements (Versluys et al. 2009).

The pneumatic powered prosthesis adhered to the following operating sequence. Heel contact is first acquired by footswitch sensor, and then the prosthesis reaches a 10° dorsiflexion angular threshold. With the angular threshold obtained, the posterior pleated pneumatic artificial muscles are pressurized to 1.5×10^5 Pascal. This pressure rating was sufficient for generating 100 Nm of plantar flexion torque based on the mass of the test subject. The pressurization of the posterior pleated pneumatic artificial muscles corresponds with the depressurization of the anterior pleated pneumatic artificial muscle to zero. Following toe-off subphase of stance the anterior pleated pneumatic artificial muscle is pressurized which mitigates the foot drop. Then all pleated pneumatic artificial muscles are reset to their gauge pressure for another gait cycle (Versluys et al. 2009).

Preliminary testing and evaluation involved a single subject. The subject was tasked to walk at a self-selected velocity, which was approximately 1.3 m/s. Based on the subject specific attributes, the stiffness of the prosthesis was set to 4.76 Nm/degrees. The primary data acquired during preliminary gait analysis was regarding the pneumatically powered prosthesis, such as prosthetic ankle angle and pressure status for the pneumatic actuator (Versluys et al. 2009).

Stance phase smoothly transitioned from heel contact to midfoot contact to forefoot contact. During this process, angular states about the ankle were achieved. Following heel contact the prosthesis reached a plantar flexion angle of −2.5°. Subsequently, 10° of dorsiflexion was attained. During the terminal aspect of stance about toe-off, the plantar flexion angle of the prosthesis achieved a threshold of −12° of plantar flexion. At the −12° of plantar flexion, maximal pressure of 1.5×10^5 Pascal corresponded with a pneumatically generated 100 Nm of torque. The findings of the study implicate the realization of pleated pneumatic artificial muscles for transtibial prosthetic applications (Versluys et al. 2009).

Future evolutions are envisioned for the actuator and control system. Most notable is the design objective of developing an untethered configuration, which is possible through a compressor. The compressor would be powered by a Li-S battery pack. Other advances about the actuator level involve amending passive springs to alleviate design requirements for the pleated pneumatic artificial muscles. A more robust control system would be necessary to enable the variable ankle stiffness with corresponding variation of walking speed, which could be facilitated by the sensors evaluating gait status (Versluys et al. 2009).

Conclusion

An assortment of actuator derived powered prostheses have been presented. Each design configuration satisfies a specific objective, such as powered plantar flexion during stance phase or facilitating toe clearance during swing phase. Single actuator and dual actuator schemes are described. As miniaturization trends have progressed the dual actuator type of powered prosthesis has become increasingly feasible. The dual actuator expands the biomimetic possibilities of the powered prosthesis, since the ankle-foot complex is inherently segmented in nature. This array of powered prostheses enables people with amputation to select a powered prosthesis that optimally satisfies their lifestyle activity preferences.

References

Au SK (2007) Powered ankle-foot prosthesis for the improvement of amputee walking economy. Ph.D. dissertation, MIT, Department of Mechanical Engineering, Cambridge

Au SK, Herr H, Weber J, Martinez-Villalpando EC (2007a) Powered ankle-foot prosthesis for the improvement of amputee ambulation. Proceedings of 29th annual international conference of the IEEE EMBS, Lyon, pp 3020–3026

Au SK, Weber J, Herr H (2007b) Biomechanical design of a powered ankle-foot prosthesis. Proceedings of IEEE 10th international conference on rehabilitation robotics, Noordwijk, pp 298–303

Au S, Berniker M, Herr H (2008) Powered ankle-foot prosthesis to assist level-ground and stair-descent gaits. Neural Netw 21:654–666

Au SK, Weber J, Herr H (2009) Powered ankle-foot prosthesis improves walking metabolic economy. IEEE Trans Robot 25:51–66

Bellman RD, Holgate MA, Sugar TG (2008) SPARKy 3: design of an active robotic ankle prosthesis with two actuated degrees of freedom using regenerative kinetics. Proceedings of 2nd IEEE RAS & EMBS international conference on biomedical robotics and biomechatronics (BioRob), Scottsdale, pp 511–516

BiOM. www.biom.com; www.bionxmed.com

Burgess EM, Poggi DL, Hittenberger DA, Zettl JH, Moeller DE, Carpenter KL, Forsgren SM (1985) Development and preliminary evaluation of the VA Seattle foot. J Rehabil Res Dev 22: 75–84

Cherelle P, Matthys A, Grosu V, Vanderborght B, Lefeber, D (2012) The AMP-foot 2.0: mimicking intact ankle behavior with a powered transtibial prosthesis. Proceedings of 4th IEEE RAS & EMBS international conference on biomedical robotics and biomechatronics (BioRob), Rome, pp 544–549

Darter BJ, Wilken JM (2014) Energetic consequences of using a prosthesis with adaptive ankle motion during slope walking in persons with a transtibial amputation. Prosthet Orthot Int 38: 5–11

Fradet L, Alimusaj M, Braatz F, Wolf SI (2010) Biomechanical analysis of ramp ambulation of transtibial amputees with an adaptive ankle foot system. Gait Posture 32:191–198

Gates DH, Aldridge JM, Wilken JM (2013) Kinematic comparison of walking on uneven ground using powered and unpowered prostheses. Clin Biomech 28:467–472

Hitt J, Merlo J, Johnston J, Holgate M, Boehler A, Hollander K, Sugar T (2010) Bionic running for unilateral transtibial military amputees. Military Academy West Point, 1–8

Holgate MA, Hitt JK, Bellman RD, Sugar TG, Hollander KW (2008) The SPARKy (Spring Ankle with Regenerative kinetics) project: choosing a DC motor based actuation method. Proceedings of 2nd IEEE RAS & EMBS international conference on biomedical robotics and biomechatronics (BioRob), Scottsdale, pp 163–168

Holgate MA, Sugar TG, Böhler AW (2009) A novel control algorithm for wearable robotics using phase plane invariants. Proceedings of IEEE international conference on robotics and automation (ICRA), Kobe, pp 3845–3850

Hollander KW, Sugar TG, Herring DE (2005) adjustable robotic tendon using a 'Jack Spring'™. Proceedings of 9th international conference on rehabilitation robotics (ICORR 2005), Chicago, pp 113–118

LeMoyne R (2015) Advances regarding powered prosthesis for transtibial amputation. J Mech Med Biol 15:1–34

Okita N, Meyers SA, Challis JH, Sharkey NA (2009) An objective evaluation of a segmented foot model. Gait Posture 30:27–34

Ossur. http://www.ossur.com

Pratt GA, Williamson MM (1995) Series elastic actuators. Proceedings of IEEE international conference on intelligent robots and systems 95. 'Human Robot Interaction and Cooperative Robots', Pittsburgh, pp 399–406

Suzuki R, Sawada T, Kobayashi N, Hofer EP (2011) Control method for powered ankle prosthesis via internal model control design. Proceedings of IEEE international conference on mechatronics and automation (ICMA), Beijing, pp 237–242

van Oort G, Carloni R, Borgerink DJ, Stramigioli S (2011) An energy efficient knee locking mechanism for a dynamically walking robot. Proceedings of IEEE international conference on Robotics and Automation (ICRA), Shanghai, pp 2003–2008

Versluys R, Lenaerts G, Van Damme M, Jonkers I, Desomer A, Vanderborght B, Peeraer L, Van der Perre G, Lefeber D (2009) Successful preliminary walking experiments on a transtibial amputee fitted with a powered prosthesis. Prosthet Orthot Int 33:368–377

Wilson AB Jr (1963) Prosthetics and orthotics research in the United States. Orthop Prosthet Appl J 17:152–160

Winter DA (1983) Energy generation and absorption at the ankle and knee during fast, natural, and slow cadences. Clin Orthop Relat Res 175:147–154

Winter DA, Sienko SE (1988) Biomechanics of below-knee amputee gait. J Biomech 21:361–367

Yuan K, Zhu J, Wang Q, Wang L (2011) Finite-state control of powered below-knee prosthesis with ankle and toe. Proceedings of 18th international federation of automatic control (IFAC) world congress, Milan, pp 2865–2870
Zhu J, Wang Q, Wang L (2010) PANTOE 1: biomechanical design of powered ankle-foot prosthesis with compliant joints and segmented foot. Proceedings of IEEE/ASME international conference on advanced intelligent mechatronics (AIM), Montréal, pp 31–36
Zhu J, Wang Q, Wang L (2014) On the design of a powered transtibial prosthesis with stiffness adaptable ankle and toe joints. IEEE Trans Ind Electron 61:4797–4807
Zlatnik D, Steiner B, Schweitzer G (2002) Finite-state control of a trans-femoral (TF) prosthesis. IEEE Trans Control Syst Technol 10:408–420

Chapter 9
The MIT Inspired Powered Prosthesis Leading to the Commercialized BiOM Powered Prosthesis, a Precedence in Transtibial Prosthetic Technology

Abstract From the research laboratories of MIT a powered prosthesis has been progressively evolved. These endeavors have led to the commercialized BiOM powered prosthesis, which constitutes a paradigm shift in available powered prostheses. The powered prosthesis satisfies a multitude of design objectives for providing a considerably biomimetic device that emulates the features of the ankle-foot complex. The key aspect of the powered prosthesis from a mechanical perspective is the series elastic actuator. The series elastic actuator regulates prosthetic ankle stiffness during preliminary stance and generates powered plantar flexion at the terminal aspect of stance. A unidirectional parallel spring facilitates actuator properties. The elastic features of the prosthetic foot aspect augment energy storage and return characteristics. A control architecture represented by a finite state controller regulates the status of the powered prosthesis. The architecture is comprised of stance and swing phase, which are further subdivided into respective subphases. A considerable amount of testing and evaluation has been applied to this format of powered prosthesis. Gait analysis experimentation contrasted to conventional passive prostheses reveals improvements in metabolic economy, increased preferred walking velocity, gait biomechanics, and adaptive capability for real-life terrain scenarios. The MIT inspired powered prosthesis leading to the BiOM powered prosthesis is envisioned to provide considerable advancement regarding quality of life opportunities for people with transtibial amputation.

Keywords Powered prosthesis • Design evolution • BiOM powered prosthesis • Biomimetic • Series elastic actuator

9.1 Introduction

The BiOM powered prosthesis constitutes a highly novel paradigm shift regarding the evolution of powered prostheses. Intrinsic features are the capacity to provide bionic propulsion through a series elastic actuator integrated into the prosthetic system. The current version enables multiple claimed utilities:

- A relatively more natural gait
- Comparable energy expenditure to a non-amputee

R. LeMoyne, *Advances for Prosthetic Technology*,
DOI 10.1007/978-4-431-55816-3_9

- The capacity to better traverse uneven terrain
- Tuning of parameters to individualize the gait cycle
- Amelioration of mechanisms that may lead to chronic degenerative morbidities
- Augmented mobility for greater opportunity for autonomy (BiOM)

This fascinating and game changing powered prosthesis has been the topic of numerous advanced research publications. The origins of the BiOM powered prosthesis derive from the research laboratories of Massachusetts Institute of Technology (MIT). In particular the research laboratory of Dr. Herr has provided an instrumental basis for the innovative evolution of the powered prosthesis (LeMoyne 2015). Because of the considerable presence of the MIT inspired powered prosthesis, which led to the BiOM, powered prosthesis an entire chapter is allocated to the research, development, testing, and evaluation that enabled this class of prosthesis.

9.2 Design Objectives for the MIT Inspired Powered Prosthesis

Design objectives were established as a foundation for the progressive evolution of the MIT inspired powered prosthesis. The following design objectives were established to consolidate the research, development, testing, and evaluation of the powered prosthesis to a well-defined challenge:

- The mass and volumetric constraints should encompass the relative scope of an intact lower limb. An approximation of roughly 18 cm from the ground to the prosthetic adapter was incorporated. The preferable mass of the powered prosthesis was scaled as a percentage of the total body mass, which was estimated about 2.5 %.
- The actuator should have torque-speed capabilities representative of a performance envelop for the human ankle respective of gait. The human ankle was characterized with a peak velocity of 3.6 rad/s, body mass normalized torque of 1.6 Nm/kg, and body mass normalized power of 3 W/kg.
- The powered prosthesis, especially the actuator, should be shock tolerant with respect to the cyclical loading imparted by stance initiation. The capacity exhibit shock tolerance is critical for a robust design, in particular highly relevant to the considerably cyclical nature of gait.
- The torque bandwidth generated by the actuator should satisfy the power spectrum respective of stance phase for human ankle torque. The torque bandwidth is characterized in terms of the frequency range that represents 70 % of the signal power.
- Respective of stance phase, the powered prosthesis should modulate stiffness. In general, an average stiffness about the ankle-foot complex is approximately 8 Nm/rad/kg normalized to unit body mass.

- Upon the terminal aspect of stance phase the powered prosthesis should contribute positive work to the gait cycle. The targeted work provided to the gait cycle through powered plantar flexion of the ankle-foot complex is established at about 0.21 J/kg, which was normalized on the basis of unit body mass.
- The powered prosthesis should regulate joint position for the swing phase of the gait cycle.

These well established design objectives were realized over the course of years of dedicated research, development, testing, and evaluation (Au et al. 2007a, b; Au 2007; Au and Herr 2008; LeMoyne 2015).

In the timeframe of 2007 the MIT powered prosthesis was comprised of five major subsystems/components:

- Three components enabling the series elastic actuator
  - A high power DC motor was incorporated through a Maxon (RE-40) 150 W brushed motor.
  - Linkage through a mechanical transmission using a 3 mm pitch linear ballscrew applying a 1.7:1 ratio timing belt drive transmission constituted the drive train for translating actuation about the motor. The ballscrew translational displacement produces angular rotation for the prosthetic ankle joint though in conjunction with the series springs that corresponds with a moment arm of 0.0375 m (3.75 cm).
  - A series spring with a spring constant of 1200 kN/m facilitated the appropriate force bandwidth requirements.
- Two other components augmenting elasticity for the prosthetic design
  - The unidirectional parallel spring was selected to have a spring stiffness of 770 kN/m with a correlated moment arm of 0.022 m (2.2 cm).
  - A prosthetic foot incorporating a carbon composite leaf spring that was represented through a Flex-Foot LP Vari-Flex.

These subsystems/components serve a highly synergistic and integral role with the satisfaction of the design objectives from a mechanical perspective (Au et al. 2007a).

The series elastic actuator constitutes the predominant source of torque for the generating positive work to the gait cycle during terminal stance phase. Prior to terminal stance phase at the controlled plantar flexion and controlled dorsiflexion aspects the series elastic actuator regulates stiffness about the prosthetic ankle joint. The series elastic actuator monitors force control through the proportion of the series spring compression. The force generated by the series elastic actuator can be derived based on the spring displacement through the integration of a linear potentiometer (Au et al. 2007a). The presence of the series spring provides the powered prosthesis with shock tolerance (Au and Herr 2008). The series elastic actuator establishes force control in a biomimetic manner, similar to the muscle spindles positioned near musculature of the human body (LeMoyne et al. 2011; LeMoyne 2015).

The amalgamation of a parallel spring is applied to alleviate constraints on the series elastic actuator imperative for sustained walking. The parallel spring is unidirectional by design for mitigating toe strike with the ground during the swing phase. The parallel spring is actively engaged to provide stiffness when the ankle angle exceeds a threshold of zero degrees. The presence of the parallel spring improves the force bandwidth to a level of a representative ankle-foot complex (Au et al. 2007a; Au and Herr 2008; LeMoyne 2015). The force bandwidth is a major parameter for a biomimetic powered prosthesis. Force bandwidth signifies the responsiveness of an actuator to apply a desired force (Robinson 2000; LeMoyne 2015).

The other passive aspect of the MIT powered prosthesis is the carbon composite leaf spring, which is conceptually similar to a passive prosthesis enabling partial energy return. There are two advantages to incorporating the leaf spring foot during stance initiation: shock absorption and associated energy absorption. A fraction of the stored elastic energy is released at the terminal phase of stance (Au et al. 2007a).

The series elastic actuator represents a paradigm shift for the technology capabilities of biped robotics (Bekey 2005). This type of actuator facilitates the development of a new class of available powered prosthesis (LeMoyne 2015). The inherent advantages of the series elastic actuator involve features, such as lower reflected inertia, improved shock tolerance, and energy storage, which may alleviate power constraints for the associated battery (Pratt and Williamson 1995).

Another benefit is in the context of the control architecture. The series elasticity improves force control, as this issue becomes associated to the subject of position control. These actuator level benefits are concealed from perceptivity of the control level (Pratt and Williamson 1995).

9.3 Control Architecture

The selection of the control architecture constitutes a major aspect in the design cycle for the development of the powered prosthesis. A pertinent version of the finite state machine was incorporated for the MIT inspired powered prosthesis. In consideration the fluid nature of gait, the finite state controller was developed to acquire status of gait phases and their respective subphases (Au et al. 2007a, 2008).

Three primary variables provided acuity to the finite state controller:

- Joint torque
- Angle of the ankle joint
- Contact status respective of the heel and toe aspects of the powered prosthesis

Six force transducers evaluated the contact status about the prosthetic aspects of the heel and toe. Four force transducers were positioned proximal to the forefoot of the powered prosthesis, and two force transducers were localized about the heel section of the powered prosthesis. An encoder positioned at the ankle joint measured the angle of the ankle joint. Joint torque was acquired as a function of the linear spring potentiometer determined joint torque (Au et al. 2007a, 2008).

For the finite state control system gait is subdivided into two phases: stance phase and swing phase. Both phases are further portioned into three subphases. This control architecture enables a computational resemblance of human gait (Au et al. 2007a).

The stance phase for the finite state control system consists of three subphases presented in sequence:

- Controlled plantar flexion
- Controlled dorsiflexion
- Powered plantar flexion

The controlled plantar flexion represents the preliminary aspect of stance phase. It is comprised of heel-strike to mid-stance. During this subphase the powered prosthesis produces a joint stiffness (K_{CP}). The following subphase involves controlled dorsiflexion, which occurs between mid-stance to powered plantar flexion or toe-off. This subphase consists of a stiffness for the prosthetic ankle joint (K_{CD}). In order for the powered plantar flexion subphase to engage the measured ankle torque should exceed a prescribed threshold (τ_{PP}). The powered plantar flexion provides a constant actuator generated torque offset ($\Delta\tau$) that is superimposed respective of the stiffness for controlled dorsiflexion (K_{CD}). In the event that the torque threshold is not exceeded the controlled dorsiflexion state persists for the control architecture (Au et al. 2007a).

As summarized in the control architecture for stance phase, there are four unique parameters that characterize the performance of stance: K_{CP}, K_{CD}, τ_{PP}, and $\Delta\tau$. The torque-offset parameter ($\Delta\tau$) represents work performed by the prosthetic ankle during the terminal aspect of stance. These four parameters that regulate the characteristics of stance phase are experimentally tuned with consideration of the subject's personal preference (Au et al. 2007a).

The control architecture for the swing phase is segmented into three aspects:

- Swing 1
- Swing 2
- Swing 3

The design of the swing control architecture facilitates smooth above ground clearance of the entire ankle-foot complex. The swing 1 state is governed by a temporal threshold (t_H), which represents the duration of swing 1 state from toe-off to t_H. During swing 1 state the powered prosthesis reorients to a predetermined angular position (θ_{toeoff}). This angular orientation serves the role of providing toe-clearance. After swing 1 state completes the swing 2 state continues until the powered prosthesis achieves a foot orientation equivalent to the default equilibrium ($\theta_d = 0$). Upon satisfying the default equilibrium swing 3 state initiates and terminates at the initial contact of stance (heel strike). The powered prosthesis is then reset to a joint stiffness (K_{CP}) (Au et al. 2007a).

The transition from state to state is identified based on the status of four significant parameters. Foot switches acquire status of heel and toe contact of the powered prosthesis. The ankle angle is evaluated through the application of an ankle joint encoder. The applied level of joint torque is ascertained based on the feedback of a linear spring potentiometer. Preliminary testing and evaluation of the powered prosthesis developed at MIT compared to conventional prostheses with passive elasticity reveal improvements in metabolic economy for walking (Au et al. 2007a).

9.4 Progressive Advances for the MIT Inspired Powered Prosthesis

Present variations of the MIT inspired powered prosthesis are referred to as a bionic prosthesis, which characterizes the progressive evolution to achieve the objective of truly emulating the properties of the ankle-foot complex. In general the global design features are retained. The bionic prosthesis has amended components with improved performance capabilities. Passive and active components have been applied to the bionic prosthesis for optimal utility, such as the generation of mechanized work about the ankle joint during the stance phase of gait (Au and Herr 2008; Eilenberg et al. 2010; Markowitz et al. 2011; Herr and Grabowski 2012). An advance of the MIT inspired powered prosthesis applied enhanced modeling of the reflex scheme and Hill muscle model (Eilenberg et al. 2010; Markowitz et al. 2011).

The series elastic actuator is capable of providing positive and negative work. The series elastic actuator is comprised of three primary components: motor, transmission, and leaf spring. A Maxon EC-Powermax 30 that incorporates a 200 W DC brushless motor provides the actuator generated the torque. The transmission converts rotational movement to linear displacement. This is achieved through a ball-screw transmission (Nook 14 × 3 mm). The incorporation of the leaf consisting of carbon composite advances actuator efficiency, which is aligned in series. The leaf spring enables energy storage and release (Herr and Grabowski 2012).

The bionic prosthesis is comprised of two other passive energy storage components. The foot aspect is designed of carbon-composite. A parallel unidirectional leaf spring is aligned in parallel with the series elastic actuator. The parallel unidirectional leaf spring is disengaged with the bionic prosthesis for angles that exceed the threshold of 90°. For angular orientations below 90° the parallel unidirectional leaf spring is capable of storing and releasing energy (Herr and Grabowski 2012).

The aggregate mass of the bionic prosthesis is on the scale of 2 kg, which is representative for a 80 kg person. Encased within the bionic prosthesis is the electronics package. Relative to the electric energy consumed the prosthesis is 67 % efficient with regards to the net positive work generated during stance. A 0.22 kg lithium-polymer rechargeable battery constitutes the power source. In excess of the general number of steps a person with an amputation takes within the scope of a day the bionic prosthesis can provide 4000 to 5000 steps (Herr and Grabowski 2012).

The bionic prosthesis integrates a real time wireless communication package. This communication package permits the user with the opportunity to modify power delivery and ankle stiffness in real time to the user's optimal preference (Herr and Grabowski 2012). The communication and control capabilities are coordinated through an integrated microcontroller. A motor controller regulates speed and computational load requirements for the brushless motor (Eilenberg et al. 2010; Herr and Grabowski 2012).

The temporal and magnitude aspects of power delivery are modulated through the application of an array of sensors integrated into the bionic prosthesis. Multiple feedback signal pathways are enabled through encoders proximal to the ankle joint and motor shaft. The sensor package also applies a 6-degree of freedom inertial measurement unit that is comprised of three accelerometers and three rate gyroscopes. With an increase in detected torque at the ankle joint of the bionic prosthesis an increase in actuator generated torque during the terminal aspect of stance phase can be commenced. In essence an increase in self-determined walking velocity could by complimented with amplified net positive work from the bionic prosthesis. The sensor array also permits the regulation of ankle torque during stance phase for gait (Herr and Grabowski 2012).

9.5 Testing and Evaluation of the MIT Inspired Powered Prosthesis and BiOM

The MIT inspired powered prosthesis and its commercialized counterpart the BiOM powered prosthesis have both undergone extensive testing and evaluation. The desire to notably advance the quality of life is the primary ambition for the developers of the powered prosthesis. The powered prosthesis is envisioned to provide benefit to gait parameters primarily as a consequence of generating actuator derived powered plantar flexion during the terminal aspect of the stance phase. Two of the most apparent parameters influencing a person with an amputation's quality of life are metabolic cost reduction while walking and amplified self-selected gait velocity from the augment of powered plantar flexion relative to conventional passive prostheses (LeMoyne 2015).

Testing and evaluation has placed an emphasis on the metabolic economy during gait. The powered prosthesis has been contrasted relative to the standard passive elastic prosthesis. The powered prosthesis logically provides enhanced metabolic economy for walking, since it produces mechanized powered plantar flexion as opposed to only a fraction of elastically conserved energy. Experimentation involved subjects walking with to conventional passive-elastic prosthesis compared to the powered prosthesis. The findings exhibited that metabolic cost of transport measured as a function of oxygen consumption was reduced while using the powered prosthesis relative to the passive prosthesis (Au et al. 2007a, 2009).

Eilenberg et al. amended a Hill muscle model to the control architecture of their experimental power prosthesis. The neuromuscular inspired control architecture was projected to enable natural adaptive characteristics as opposed to control schemes that rely on prescribed ankle torque profiles. Another feature of the neuromuscular inspired control architecture is the integration of a positive force feedback reflex scheme. Testing and evaluation of the experimental powered prosthesis pertained to three walking scenarios:

- Level ground
- Ramp ascent
- Ramp descent

The biomechanics of the gait cycle were measured through conventional gait analysis equipment; such as a motion capture system and two staggered force plates. The neuromuscular inspired control architecture benefited the experimental powered prosthesis. Adaptive modulation of generated torque was demonstrated in the context of walking condition. The research emphasized the significance of neuromuscular control systems improving prosthetic adaptation with regards to diverse terrain surfaces (Eilenberg et al. 2010).

People with transtibial amputation that walk with a conventional prosthesis typically experience amplified metabolic demands, which associate with diminished walking speeds, presumably due to a lack of powered plantar flexion during stance phase of gait (Waters et al. 1976; Hsu et al. 2006; Herr and Grabowski 2012; LeMoyne 2015). Herr and Grabowski conducted research focusing on the capacity of the powered prosthesis to mitigate adverse biomechanics during gait and reduce metabolic demands. The experiment applied an assortment of gait analysis devices. A portable metabolic analysis system evaluated metabolic loads induced during walking. The ground reaction force was measured by force plates. Gait velocity was acquired through a motion analysis system (Herr and Grabowski 2012).

By comparison to the conventional passive elastic prosthesis the powered prosthesis provided its user with a reduction in metabolic cost during gait. The subjects walking with the powered prosthesis trended away from the less efficient metabolic cost of transport as a function of gait velocity relationship for passive prosthesis and toward a more efficient metabolic cost of transport as a function of gait velocity relationship for people without amputation. The preferred walking velocity in general provides the metabolic cost of transport optimal, which is the minimum for the metabolic cost of transport as a function of gait velocity relationship. The preferred walking velocity for people with amputation using the powered prosthesis shifted to nearly the equivalence of the preferred waking velocity for people without amputation. Representing the trailing leg the powered prosthesis produced positive work that was similar to people without amputation. Collision work regarding the intact leg was comparable to people without amputation (Herr and Grabowski 2012).

Comparable results were provide by Mancinelli et al. in terms of reduced oxygen consumption and amplified power generation during the terminal aspect of stance phase (Mancinelli et al. 2011). Another research experiment further revealed that the powered prosthesis compared to a standard prosthesis trended to a higher walking velocity respective of the minimal cost of metabolic transport (Herr and Grabowski 2010). A similar themed study determined significant difference for the powered prosthesis compared to a conventional prosthesis with regards to maximum joint power (Grabowski et al. 2011).

The BiOM powered prosthesis has been proposed to mitigate kinetic loading of the intact leg during gait. Hill and Herr developed an experiment to contrast the conventional passive prosthesis to the BiOM powered prosthesis with respective to the kinetic load imparted on the intact leg. Parameters of the BiOM were tuned by wireless connectivity through Bluetooth using an Android tablet. Kinetic and kinematic biomechanical data was quantified through the application of a pressure sensor mounted to a shoe for the biological foot, force plate, and an opto-electronic motion capture system. Relative to the conventional passive prosthesis the BiOM powered prosthesis provided a reduction in negative leading-leg transition work. Positive work generated by the trailing leg transition was considerable greater for the BiOM powered prosthesis relative to the standard powered prosthesis (Hill and Herr 2013). Chronically degenerative morbidities, such as knee osteoarthritis, have been correlated with the magnitude of external adduction moment regarding the knee, in terms of severity and progression (Mündermann et al. 2005; Morgenroth et al. 2011; Morgenroth et al. 2012; Hill and Herr 2013).

Grabowski and D'Andrea investigated the influence of influence of the BiOM powered prosthesis with regards to kinetic loading for the intact leg. Their experimental apparatus consisted of force plates and a motion analysis system. A conventional passive prosthesis was contrasted to the BiOM powered prosthesis. Respective of the intact leg ground reaction force rate, first peak ground reaction force, first peak external adduction moment about the knee, and the rate for the external adduction moment about the knee displayed relatively decreasing trends for the BiOM powered prosthesis. An advanced powered prosthesis, such as the BiOM powered prosthesis, could ameliorate the risk of developing knee osteoarthritis with reduced kinetic loading for the intact leg (Grabowski and D'Andrea 2013).

The BiOM powered prosthesis is highly relevant to real-life scenarios, such as stair ascent. Optoelectronic motion capture system and force plates to quantify the biomechanical features during stair ascent. Although subjects persisted to apply a hip strategy during stair ascent, the BiOM powered prosthesis demonstrated increased range of motion for the ankle and improved power during ascent by comparison to traditional prosthesis with passive elasticity (Aldridge et al. 2012).

The BiOM powered prosthesis was compared to the passive energy storage return prosthesis while traversing a loose rock surface. Gait kinematics were acquired through a motion capture system. Subjects exhibited improvement for ankle joint kinematics and increased self-selected walking speed (Gates et al. 2013).

Markowitz et al. integrated a neuromuscular model in to the powered prosthesis for more adaptive user-determined adjustments to gait cycle, such as increasing work about the prosthetic ankle in response to increased walking speed. The neuromuscular model applied a reflex feedback system and the Hill muscle model. Average walking speed was calculated based on a fixed distance using a stopwatch. The control architecture with a neuromuscular model featured adaptive characteristics with ankle work increasing with walking speed (Markowitz et al. 2011).

Conclusion

MIT has progressively evolved a powered prosthesis from its research laboratories to a commercialized version known as the BiOM powered prosthesis. The design strategy represents a paradigm shift for the capabilities of the transtibial powered prosthesis. The powered prosthesis provides considerably realistic emulation of the ankle-foot complex during gait by satisfying a series of well considered design objectives. Foundational to the success of this type of powered prosthesis from a mechanical perspective is the series elastic actuator. During the initial segment of stance the series elastic actuator adjusts stiffness about the prosthetic ankle. At terminal stance powered plantar flexion is mechanically generated. The properties of the series elastic actuator are facilitated through a unidirectional parallel spring. Energy return capabilities are advanced through a prosthetic foot with elastic properties. A finite state controller comprises the control architecture, which determines status regarding stance and swing phase inclusive of respective subphases. The capacity of this type of powered prosthesis has been established with a considerable amount of testing and evaluation. Relative to conventional passive prostheses, the MIT inspired powered prosthesis and BiOM powered prosthesis demonstrate enhanced metabolic economy, increased preferred walking velocity, improved gait biomechanics, and adaptive capability for real-life terrain scenarios through the application of gait analysis systems. The MIT inspired powered prosthesis and BiOM powered prosthesis are projected to deliver major improvement in consideration to quality of life opportunities for people with transtibial amputation.

References

Aldridge JM, Sturdy JT, Wilken JM (2012) Stair ascent kinematics and kinetics with a powered lower leg system following transtibial amputation. Gait Posture 36:291–295

Au SK (2007) Powered ankle-foot prosthesis for the improvement of amputee walking economy. Ph.D. dissertation, MIT, Department of Mechanical Engineering, Cambridge

Au SK, Herr HM (2008) Powered ankle-foot prosthesis. IEEE Robot Autom Mag 15:52–59

Au SK, Herr H, Weber J, Martinez-Villalpando EC (2007a) Powered ankle-foot prosthesis for the improvement of amputee ambulation. Proceedings of 29th annual international conference of the IEEE EMBS, Lyon, pp 3020–3026

Au SK, Weber J, Herr H (2007b) Biomechanical design of a powered ankle-foot prosthesis. Proceedings of IEEE 10th international conference on rehabilitation robotics, Noordwijk, pp 298–303

Au S, Berniker M, Herr H (2008) Powered ankle-foot prosthesis to assist level-ground and stair-descent gaits. Neural Netw 21:654–666

Au SK, Weber J, Herr H (2009) Powered ankle-foot prosthesis improves walking metabolic economy. IEEE Trans Robot 25:51–66

Bekey GA (2005) Autonomous robots: from biological inspiration to implementation and control. MIT Press, Cambridge

BiOM. www.biom.com; www.bionxmed.com

Eilenberg MF, Geyer H, Herr H (2010) Control of a powered ankle–foot prosthesis based on a neuromuscular model. IEEE Trans Neural Syst Rehabil Eng 18:164–173

Gates DH, Aldridge JM, Wilken JM (2013) Kinematic comparison of walking on uneven ground using powered and unpowered prostheses. Clin Biomech 28:467–472

Grabowski AM, D'Andrea S (2013) Effects of a powered ankle-foot prosthesis on kinetic loading of the unaffected leg during level-ground walking. J Neuroeng Rehabil 10:1–11

Grabowski A, D'Andrea S, Herr H (2011) Bionic leg prosthesis emulates biological ankle joint during walking. Proceedings of 35th annual meeting of the American Society of Biomechanics, Long Beach, pp 1–2

Herr HM, Grabowski AM (2010) Powered ankle-foot prosthesis improves metabolic demand of unilateral transtibial amputees during walking. Proceedings of 34th annual meeting of the American Society of Biomechanics, Providence, pp 1–2

Herr HM, Grabowski AM (2012) Bionic ankle–foot prosthesis normalizes walking gait for persons with leg amputation. Proc Biol Sci 279:457–464

Hill D, Herr H (2013) Effects of a powered ankle-foot prosthesis on kinetic loading of the contralateral limb: a case series. Proceedings of IEEE 13th international conference on rehabilitation robotics, Seattle, pp 1–6

Hsu MJ, Nielsen DH, Lin-Chan SJ, Shurr D (2006) The effects of prosthetic foot design on physiologic measurements, self-selected walking velocity, and physical activity in people with transtibial amputation. Arch Phys Med Rehabil 87:123–129

LeMoyne R (2015) Advances regarding powered prosthesis for transtibial amputation. J Mech Med Biol 15:1–34

LeMoyne R, Mastroianni T, Coroian C, Grundfest W (2011) Tendon reflex and strategies for quantification, with novel methods incorporating wireless accelerometer reflex quantification devices, a perspective review. J Mech Med Biol 11:471–513

Mancinelli C, Patritti BL, Tropea P, Greenwald RM, Casler R, Herr H, Bonato P (2011) Comparing a passive-elastic and a powered prosthesis in transtibial amputees. Proceedings of 33rd annual international conference of the IEEE EMBS, Boston, pp 8255–8258

Markowitz J, Krishnaswamy P, Eilenberg MF, Endo K, Barnhart C, Herr H (2011) Speed adaptation in a powered transtibial prosthesis controlled with a neuromuscular model. Philos Trans R Soc Lond B Biol Sci 366:1621–1631

Morgenroth DC, Segal AD, Zelik KE, Czerniecki JM, Klute GK, Adamczyk PG, Orendurff MS, Hahn ME, Collins SH, Kuo AD (2011) The effect of prosthetic foot push-off on mechanical loading associated with knee osteoarthritis in lower extremity amputees. Gait Posture 34:502–507

Morgenroth DC, Gellhorn AC, Suri P (2012) Osteoarthritis in the disabled population: a mechanical perspective. PM R 4:S20–S27

Mündermann A, Dyrby CO, Andriacchi TP (2005) Secondary gait changes in patients with medial compartment knee osteoarthritis: increased load at the ankle, knee, and hip during walking. Arthritis Rheum 52:2835–2844

Pratt GA, Williamson MM (1995) Series elastic actuators. Proceedings of IEEE international conference on intelligent robots and systems 95. 'Human Robot Interaction and Cooperative Robots', Pittsburgh, pp 399–406

Robinson DW (2000) Design and analysis of series elasticity in closed-loop actuator force control. Ph.D. dissertation, MIT, Department of Mechanical Engineering, Cambridge

Waters RL, Perry J, Antonelli D, Hislop H (1976) Energy cost of walking of amputees: the influence of level of amputation. J Bone Joint Surg Am 58:42–46

Chapter 10
Future and Advanced Concepts for the Powered Prosthesis

Abstract Future and advanced concepts facilitate considerable opportunity for the powered prosthesis. Since the powered prosthesis constitutes a mechatronic system, many other trends of industry, science, and engineering are anticipated to provide technological advance on the system, subsystem, and component level. Currently powered prostheses are equipped with localized wireless connectivity, and this capability can be augmented to Internet connectivity through a smartphone or portable media device. Synergy with the Internet of Things is envisioned to substantially advance the adaptive capacity of the powered prosthesis much to the likeness of the plasticity of and intact lower limb. Remote tele-rehabilitation is projected to enable unique therapy opportunities while alleviating implied logistic constraints inherent with traditional therapy sessions. Another advanced concept is the increasing significance of 3D printing. 3D printed materials are predicted to eventually attain property characteristics, such that they could be incorporated for structural elements of the prosthesis. Image scanning techniques may be applied to emulate skeletal and cosmetic features of the intact lower leg for 3D printing. In summary many opportunities exist regarding advances for prosthetic technology.

Keywords Mechatronic system • Internet of Things • Machine learning • Localized wireless connectivity • 3D printing

10.1 Introduction

As the powered prosthesis is representative of a mechatronic system trends of advancement are anticipated for many of its supporting technologies. As specified in Chap. 7: 'Architecture of a powered prosthesis system: actuators, sensors, and control' multiple subsystems and components are foundational to the capabilities of the powered prosthesis. As these aspects are also likely influenced by other industries their evolutionary pathways will probably be enhanced by factors outside of the powered prosthetic sphere of influence.

As an example consider the accelerometer which provides sensory feedback regarding spatial representation. Many decades ago accelerometers were proposed for the role of gait analysis. However at that time accelerometers were not sufficiently developed for actual implementation for human gait analysis. Rather than

R. LeMoyne, *Advances for Prosthetic Technology*,
DOI 10.1007/978-4-431-55816-3_10

being progressively evolved through the influence of the biomedical community, accelerometer devices experienced considerable advance from the influence of the automotive industry. Progressive improvements in miniaturization lead to the accelerometer being viable for eventual human gait analysis (LeMoyne et al. 2008, 2009).

This scenario is highly likely for the technology evolution of powered prosthesis systems. Outside influences will probably drive the advancement of foundational aspects for the powered prosthesis. A notable feature inherent with current powered prostheses is the capability for wirelessly connectivity in a local context (LeMoyne 2015; BiOM). This observation synergizes the powered prosthesis with a pathway of tremendous capability known as the Internet of Things.

10.2 The Internet of Things and 3D Printing Regarding the Powered Prosthesis

The Internet of Things essentially facilitates the connectivity of devices and sensors to the Internet. Three primary categories encompass automotive applications, home monitoring, and health status tracking (Swan 2012). With localized wireless connectivity to a smartphone a powered prosthesis could feasibly be integrated with the Internet of Things.

In principle LeMoyne et al. during 2014 achieved a preliminary representation of the Internet of Things for prosthetic applications. A 3D printed adapter enables a smartphone to be mounted to a passive prosthesis. The smartphone was equipped with a software platform to function as a wireless accelerometer with Internet connectivity through email (LeMoyne et al. 2014). The sensor platforms of smartphones and portable media devices have been demonstrated to monitor subject health status with Internet connectivity (LeMoyne and Mastroianni 2015).

The telemetry of the powered prosthesis could be locally connected by wireless transmission to a smartphone. The smartphone would be capable of connecting the telemetry stream to Internet resources. Post-processing can be achieved with machine learning classification, essentially facilitating prognostic acuity of the person using the powered prosthesis.

Preliminary demonstration of machine learning classification has been demonstrated for the scope of prosthetic applications. Considerable classification accuracy has been achieved with regards to distinguishing between a subject using a passive prosthesis and powered prosthesis through the application of a support vector machine and a conventional gait analysis system (LeMoyne et al. 2015). Wireless accelerometers have been successfully advocated as more advanced relative to conventional gait analysis equipment, and smartphones and portable media devices readily access the Internet through email (LeMoyne et al. 2008, LeMoyne and Mastroianni 2015).

Access to the Internet of Things with effectively diagnostic and prognostic machine learning applications would facilitate a person with an amputation with optimal adaptability. As noted in Chap. 2 'Ankle-foot complex and the fundamental aspects of gait' the ankle-foot complex is highly adaptive with the capacity to exhibit plasticity throughout a person's modifications to lifestyle preferences. Although even a powered prosthesis in general is not nearly as robustly adaptive as an intact ankle-foot complex, the association with the Internet of Things could greatly facilitate robust adaptive capacity.

Upon machine learning applications distinguishing a modification in activity patterns based on data acquired from the telemetry of the powered prosthesis an efficient course of action could be determined. For example, a new software platform could be uploaded to the powered prosthetic to more optimally accommodate the person with an amputation. In consideration of the supporting hardware the enables the powered prosthesis, a local prosthetist could be contacted for proactively providing an appropriate hardware upgrade. Given the global reach of the Internet, a person with amputation could engage in tele-rehabilitation far remote from the resources of the clinical environment, which could alleviate logistic resources.

Another topic associated with logistic efficiency is the subject of 3D printing. 3D printing is becoming increasingly relevant toward prosthetic applications. Custom made prosthetic components can be uniquely tailored to the person with amputation (Army; Natick).

Future extrapolations anticipate that 3D printing capabilities will probably improve substantially. As 3D printing material become more durable structural elements, such as the pylon and energy absorbing foot, may be derived from 3D prints. With the eventual synergy of radiology and highly robust 3D printing the intact lower limb's skeletal structure could be replicated for a highly biomimetic powered prosthesis system. Actual bone and joint relationships based on the intact leg could be represented in the powered prosthesis possibly enabling considerable energy absorption capacity. Cosmetic emulation of the intact leg could be highly developed through an image scan of the intact leg.

Conclusion

In summary future evolutionary trends for the powered prosthesis are predicted to be driven by peripherally associated industries. Current powered prostheses display wireless characteristics, which can relate them to the Internet of Things. The Internet of Things with prognostic machine learning is anticipated to enable highly responsive adaptation to any desired modifications with regards to lifestyle activities. 3D printing is envisioned to further facilitate a highly personalized experience for people with amputation and their unique preferences.

References

Army. http://www.army.mil/article/88464/Army_researchers_use_cutting_edge_3D_printers/

BiOM. www.biom.com; www.bionxmed.com

LeMoyne R (2015) Advances regarding powered prosthesis for transtibial amputation. J Mech Med Biol 15:1–34

LeMoyne R, Mastroianni T (2015) Use of smartphones and portable media devices for quantifying human movement characteristics of gait, tendon reflex response, and Parkinson's disease hand tremor, chap 23. In: Rasooly A, Herold KE (eds) Mobile health technologies: methods and protocols. Springer, New York

LeMoyne R, Coroian C, Mastroianni T, Grundfest W (2008) Accelerometers for quantification of gait and movement disorders: a perspective review. J Mech Med Biol 8:137–152

LeMoyne R, Coroian C, Mastroianni T, Opalinski P, Cozza M, Grundfest W (2009) The merits of artificial proprioception, with applications in biofeedback gait rehabilitation concepts and movement disorder characterization, chap 10. In: de Barros Mello CA (ed) Biomedical engineering. Intech, Vienna

LeMoyne R, Mastroianni T, Montoya K (2014) Implementation of a smartphone for evaluating gait characteristics of a trans-tibial prosthesis. Proceedings of 36th annual international conference of the IEEE EMBS, Chicago, pp 3674–3677

LeMoyne R, Mastroianni T, Hessel A, Nishikawa K (2015) Implementation of machine learning for classifying prosthesis type through conventional gait analysis. Proceedings of 37th annual international conference of the IEEE EMBS, Milan, pp 202–205

Natick. http://www.army.mil/article/119962/Natick_s__model__employee/

Swan M (2012) Sensor mania! the internet of things, wearable computing, objective metrics, and the quantified self 2.0. J Sens Actuator Netw 1:217–253

Biography

Dr. Robert LeMoyne is currently serving as a Post-Doctoral Scholar for Northern Arizona University. At Northern Arizona University he is researching advanced technology for transtibial powered prosthesis applications. He earned his PhD in Biomedical Engineering from University of California Los Angeles (UCLA) during 2010. From 2010 to 2012 he served Sandia National Laboratories, and since 2013 he has been serving Northern Arizona University. From a biomedical engineering perspective his research interests emphasize prosthetic technologies, machine learning applications, and mobile platforms, such as through smartphones and portable media devices, for accessing health status.

R. LeMoyne, *Advances for Prosthetic Technology*,
DOI 10.1007/978-4-431-55816-3

Index

R. LeMoyne, *Advances for Prosthetic Technology*,
DOI 10.1007/978-4-431-55816-3

FSC
www.fsc.org
MIX
Papier | Fördert
gute Waldnutzung
FSC® C083411

Kolibri 360 GmbH
Ferdinand-Jühlke-Straße 7
99095 Erfurt, Deutschland
produktsicherheit@kolibri360.de